ePATIENT 2015

15 Surprising Trends Changing Health Care

"*A fascinating and groundbreaking look at how technology and empowered patients are fundamentally changing health care.*"

ROHIT BHARGAVA
Best Selling Author of
Likeonomics

FARD JOHNMAR
Founder of
Enspektos

ePatient 2015

15 Surprising Trends
Changing Health Care

Rohit Bhargava
Founder, Influential Marketing Group, Inc.
Author of the #1 Best Seller, *Likeonomics*

Fard Johnmar
Founder, Enspektos, LLC
Digital Health Futurist and Researcher

PUBLISHED BY IDEAPRESS PUBLISHING

IDEAPRESS PUBLISHING is a trademark of Influential Marketing Group, Inc.
ENSPEKTOS, ENMOEBIUS AND DIGIHEALTH PULSE are registered
trademarks of Enspektos, LLC

Copyright 2013/2014 by Rohit Bhargava and Fard Johnmar

Cataloging-in-Publication Data is on file with the Library of Congress

ISBN: 9781940858005

Book Cover and Interior Design by Robert Kalnitz

All Rights Reserved

PRINTED IN THE UNITED STATES OF AMERICA

First Edition: December 2013
All trademarks are the property of their respective companies.

CUSTOM PRINTING + BULK SALES
This publication is available at special discounts for bulk purchases or custom
printing. For more information, please visit www.epatient2015.com.

All URLs included in this book were current as of the printing of this publication.

Advance Praise for ePatient 2015

"Changes in our healthcare system are being driven by rapid advances in mobile platforms, health information technology, and social media. Fard Johnmar and Rohit Bhargava have monitored these trends from the start, and their book, ePatient 2015 - 15 Surprising Trends Changing Health Care, is a prescient roadmap that guides both patients and doctors as their relationships evolve."

—Kevin Pho, Founder and Editor, KevinMD.com

"The clairvoyance displayed by the authors is not only spot on, but is a welcome and disruptive shift from the current aseptic and vacuous thinking that has withheld true innovation and progress in the digital health sector. Free your mind, eliminate barriers to your success, and read this book."

—Matthew Zachary, Patient Advocate, Founder and CEO, Stupid Cancer

"ePatient 2015 is a valuable resource for digital health amateurs and experts alike. Fard and Rohit's focus on the patient as the center of the dynamic digital health world grounds their analysis of the space in a way that is both logical and incredibly relevant. The book highlights 15 trends that ultimately reflect the authors' deep understanding of the space, and serve as a shrewd guide to how technology and the social consumer are changing the face of modern health care."

— Kim Krueger, Research Analyst Health 2.0 and
Prerna Anand, Data Analyst, Health 2.0

"Fard and Rohit provide readers with a sense of what health care will be like in the near future, most notably how patients will receive much more actionable information that can help them make smart decisions about their own care, which is fundamentally different from just a few generations ago. For those in business who wonder where technology in health care will take their products, the 15 trends identified in this book can help them strategically plan for the future. Most importantly, it highlights what we believe about health care overall, that through collaboration and peer support, patients and their caregivers will receive a personalized and highly relevant care experience."

—Robert Nauman, Digital Strategist, Founder BioPharma Advisors

What's Next in Digital Health?
Find Out with enmoebius bronze

enmoebius (bronze)

Powered by the leading digital health consultancy, Enspektos, LLC, enmoebius bronze is a member-supported intelligence service featuring more than 250 reports, webinars, infographics, and more on the evolving digital health landscape. Subscribers can also access additional insights on topics covered in *ePatient 2015* and data not featured in this book.

In addition, enmoebius bronze members have exclusive access to insights and advice from digital health experts, including Fard Johnmar, co-author of *ePatient 2015*.

Join subscribers from top organizations like the Mayo Clinic on enmoebius bronze. To learn more about the service and how to start your free 10-day trial, visit:

http://digihealth.info/digihealthintel

"The real danger is not that computers will begin to think like men, but that men will begin to think like computers."

—Sydney J. Harris

FJ: To Sotheary and Alexi

RB: To empathetic innovators, with gratitude.

Contents

Prelude:
Why This Book is Like a Good Sneeze

Empowerment. Technology. Innovation. ePatients.

These are just some of the buzzwords that are frequently used in global discussions about health care. Every day there are new media reports about the failures and successes of those leading and shaping the healthcare industry while people battling illness—far removed from the public eye—are experiencing a breadth of emotions, ranging from fear to worry, confusion, and hope.

Health care is a real-time topic for all of us. As a result, many within it—doctors, patients, caregivers, and others—do not have the luxury of taking the long view or looking at events from a broader perspective. Our aim is to offer a big picture, people-oriented overview of what's next in health care.

We journey from the emerging realm of neuro-influence to the popular topic of wearable devices. We interview digital health futurists and ePatients who have launched emotion-driven global movements. And through it all, we have broadened our lens to capture a bigger view of the future. In this book, you'll learn about 15 trends that are fundamentally changing the way all of us experience health care. Pioneering technologies drive some of them. Ordinary people have sparked others when they have been inspired—or forced—to lead their peers.

By bringing these trends together, our goal was to curate and share a quantifiable and well-researched vision of the future of health care. From the beginning, we resisted the impulse to approach our work with preconceived notions; instead, we decided to fearlessly follow the stories, trends, data, and technologies we uncovered—all the while unsure of what our effort would ultimately reveal about tomorrow.

As you'll see from the original data, dozens of stories, and many interviews we include in this book, the future of health care is an exciting one. And though the portrait we paint is not entirely rosy—several of our trends focus on the negatives of innovation—our vision for the future is an optimistic and human-focused one.

As American author Robert Benchley once wrote, "A good rousing sneeze, one that tears open your collar and throws your hair into your eyes, is really one of life's sensational pleasures."

The process of writing this book was a bit like that sneeze . . . and we hope your experience reading it will be as well.

Introduction

Little Sally's Fever and Henry's Doctor Delivers Some Very Bad News

The easy place to start a book about the future of health care is with a discussion of technologies or innovations, but we'd like to take a different approach. At its core, this book is about how digital health tools will benefit, harm, enlighten, confuse, empower, disempower, and influence people today, by 2015, and beyond.

Because of this, we think you will gain a deeper appreciation for the profound technology-driven changes to come if we began by telling two fictional, but plausible stories. The first is about a little girl named Sally, whose mother is very worried about her. The second focuses on Henry, who is about to receive some very bad news from his doctor. You'll read two versions of these tales: one set in 2013 (at the time of writing this book) and the other in 2015.

2013: Sally Has a Fever and Mom Can't Sleep

The room is dark except for the red light coming from the black digital clock sitting on Martha's nightstand. It is 2:23 a.m. and Martha can't sleep. Earlier that day she had rushed home from work to pick up her three-year-old, Sally, from day care early. One of the caretakers, Heidi, had been worried because Sally was not eating well and complaining that her head hurt.

When they got home, Martha took Sally's temperature using an ear thermometer she'd purchased from the local drug store. Unfortunately, she wasn't sure what to think because when she measured Sally's right ear, the temperature read 98.9 degrees Fahrenheit. When she inserted the thermometer into her left ear, she got a reading of 102.1. And it was almost impossible to get Sally to sit still for the temperature reading anyway.

Martha had read online somewhere that a low dose of Tylenol combined with some "fluids" could help bring down Sally's fever. She decided to err on the side of caution and gave some to Sally. On the bottle, the suggested dosage said 5 ml for children 2 to 3 years old—but Sally was 3 and 10 months and a little big for her age according to those strange height and weight percentile charts she'd seen at the pediatrician's office. She wasn't sure if the 2 - 3 year old dose would be enough, but it was close to 10 p.m. and she didn't want to leave a message on her pediatrician's after-hours answering service only to wait for a callback. So she gave Sally 5 ml, fed her some soup, and put her to bed.

At midnight, Martha checked Sally's temperature. The ear thermometer didn't seem to be working very well. Each time, the right and left ears gave her different readings, sometimes as high as 103.5. Was Sally's fever getting worse? Did she have enough medicine?

Searching Google for answers was little help. Martha had read dozens of articles about fevers in children, but each provided her with conflicting advice. Some people recommended doing nothing while others said she should call her doctor.

It was now past two a.m. and Martha was frustrated and tired. "I need some answers," she thought, reaching for her cell phone. "I'm calling Dr. Mason." Getting through to the answering service, she left a voicemail and waits for a callback from Dr. Mason, or one of the other doctors in his practice who happens to be on call.

A stressful 26 minutes later, she received a callback from another doctor in Dr. Mason's practice so she explains Sally's symptoms. "When is the last time she came in?" the new doctor asks. "Last month," Martha responded, wondering why the doctor didn't already know that from her file.

The doctor tells her it's probably a cold and to watch Sally's fever to make sure it doesn't go above 104. "This is going to be a long night," Martha told herself, staring blankly at the blinking digital display on her thermometer and reaching for her TV's remote control.

2015: Sally Has a Fever and Mom's Fast Asleep

The room is completely dark except for a soft blue light coming from the Well Home mobile application sitting on Martha's nightstand. It is 2:23 a.m. and Martha is sound asleep. Earlier that day she'd rushed home from work to pick up her three-year-old Sally from day care early. One of the caregivers, Heidi, had been worried because Sally was not eating well and complaining that her head hurt. Yet, Martha wasn't lying awake tossing and turning. Why? A medical device she'd purchased a few months earlier helped her understand what was happening with her daughter and how best to manage Sally's fever.

The device she had picked up from a local store was a new medical sensing technology that could interface with her Well Home smartphone app and monitor things like blood pressure, body temperature, and more. When she arrived home from day care, she attached the sensor to Sally's forehead so that it could continuously measure her daughter's temperature, heart rate, mood, and other vital signs. The device passively took temperature readings every hour throughout the evening. Sally's temperature hovered between 100.6 and 100.9 degrees Fahrenheit.

After each reading, the device automatically connected to Martha's online family medical record to track the temperature against previous norms for Sally and other children in their local area. Just before Martha put Sally to bed, she received a text message on her mobile phone featuring a link to an article with suggestions on how to manage minor fevers like Sally's. (She'd given the sensor manufacturer permission to send her text messages containing useful health information based on data she collected with the device.) The doctor who wrote the article suggested that low-grade fevers like Sally's shouldn't be treated.

Just for final confirmation, Martha initiated a conversation with one of her pre-selected doctors who was immediately available for a face-to-face video chat via the telepresence module located on her Well Home mobile application. Martha turned the phone towards Sally so the doctor could have a look. "She looks fine, just let her get some rest," the doctor advised. "If her temperature goes above 101, you can give her a small dose of medicine. Based on her height, weight, and physical characteristics, my medical decision support tool suggests a dose of 7 ml should be about right."

Later that night, Martha's health monitor watch woke her gently with an alert that Sally's fever had increased to 101, so Martha administered the medicine, and Sally went immediately back to sleep.

After 15 minutes, Martha did too, confident that Sally would feel better in the morning.

2013: Henry Receives Some Very Bad News

Every time Henry shifted position, his chair made an annoying squeaking sound. Squeak, squeak, squeak. "Can't the hospital afford to have someone fix this chair?" he thought. Henry's physician, Dr. Thompson, was speaking but Henry wasn't listening. His mind went blank when she said, "The biopsy confirmed that you have non-small cell lung cancer." "This is not happening," thought Henry.

Dr. Thompson stopped speaking and looked at Henry for a moment. "We have a lot to discuss," she said, "but I can tell you need some time." "Here's some information about the type of cancer you have," she continued while handing over a few pamphlets and pieces of paper. "Please see the receptionist to schedule another appointment and we'll discuss your treatment options."

Henry walked out of the hospital in a daze and drove from the parking lot. "How did this happen?" he wondered. He wasn't a heavy smoker. He was pretty sure he didn't have a family history of cancer, but it was hard to be sure because he didn't really keep in touch with many of his relatives on his father's side. When he got home, his first thought was to go online to learn more. He typed the words "non-small cell lung cancer" into Google. The results were scary. The photos of other patients with similar conditions looked gruesome. And the search page featured dozens of sites and all kinds of advice on some very involved ways he could "fight back," from getting better air filters for his home to changing his diet completely. And most medical journals Henry read were incomprehensible. Even worse, lots of sites promising some type of "all-natural" cancer cure were abundant.

The "support" forums were even tougher to navigate. There seemed to be lots of conversations, but he wasn't really confident he could jump into them when no one knew him. It felt intimidating, and he was sure he didn't have hours to devote to joining some online conversation group anyway.

After a few hours, he stopped reading, put his head in his hands, and thought: "What am I going to do?"

2015: Henry Receives Some Bad (and Good) News

Every time Henry shifted position, his chair made an annoying squeaking sound. Squeak, squeak, squeak. "Couldn't the hospital afford to have someone fix this chair?" he thought. Henry's physician, Dr. Thompson was speaking, but Henry wasn't listening. His mind went blank when she said, "the biopsy confirmed that you have non-small cell lung cancer." "This is not happening," thought Henry.

Dr. Thompson stopped speaking and looked at Henry for a moment. "I know this is hard for you," she said, "but there's some information I think you should know." "Today, it's common to test cancer cells for certain genetic and molecular characteristics," she said. "We do this because we're now able to treat the disease with a scalpel rather than a hammer," she continued. "We think your cancer is the type we've found responds very well to a particular type of medication that has fewer side effects and is much more effective than standard chemotherapy."

"This won't be an easy journey," Dr. Thompson cautioned, "but cancer treatment has changed dramatically over the past few years. And, all the lifestyle and health data that you have been capturing through that device you've been wearing will help us find the course of treatment that will best fit with your level of activity and overall health."

"How did this happen—is there anything I could have done differently?" Henry wondered out loud. "A year ago, you and other members of your family gave us permission to access, share, and analyze your high-level electronic medical records and health history," Dr. Thompson said. "It looks like your cousin on your father's side also had the same condition—and the good news is that he's doing well," shared Dr. Thompson. "That's interesting," Henry said. "I heard about a cousin who had cancer, but I didn't pay more attention because we're not that close and haven't seen each other since we were kids."

"Well it looks like you may learn a lot more about him," Dr. Thompson said. "We have data on how his medicine has been performing for him, and we can send a private request to see if he would be willing to share this information with you."

"So what should I do now?" asked Henry. "Well, doctors aren't just prescribing medications these days," replied Dr. Thompson. "I'm going to write you a prescription for a free application you can download to your smartphone. It's been tested and we know it has high quality information. You can also use it to connect with others who have non-small cell lung cancer. I'd also like you to use the app to track how you're feeling, how your medications are performing, and other important details. The good news is, it will sync with the wristband I see you're already wearing—and use all your past data to help us track your progress. The information you provide using the app will be automatically and securely sent to me, as well as added to your medical record. It will also help make your visits with me more productive. Here's information on where you can go to download the app. Please see the receptionist to schedule another appointment."

Henry left the hospital and drove out of the parking lot feeling worried but hopeful, too. After arriving home, he immediately downloaded the mobile application his doctor prescribed. The app provided him with a list of recommended online resources about non-small cell lung cancer.

He turned on the computer and went online to start reading more about his condition. Thirty minutes later, he received a text alert from the app. It was another patient, Pablo, who had been automatically paired with him as a "mentor" to help him through the first days of the disease. Pablo offered to give him a call that evening. Henry immediately accepted Pablo's invitation. An hour later, he received a secure message from his cousin accepting the request to share medical data and offering to speak by phone that weekend.

"This won't be easy," he thought, getting ready to respond to his cousin, "but I think I'm going to beat this."

What These Stories Teach Us About the Transformative Role of Information and Technology in Health

What do these fictional stories illustrate? At their heart, they both have a message of hope for the future of health care that is fueled by a combination of technology advancements and empowered patients. Today, stories of empowerment are more than just fiction—thanks to trailblazers who have jumpstarted and given a face to the ePatient movement. One of the most visible is cancer survivor, Dave deBronkart, who is known to most people (and the global healthcare industry) as ePatient Dave.

ePatient Dave is considered by many to be the quintessential example of the knowledgeable and empowered patient. He believes that technology has the potential to unleash a wave of innovation in health, but only if the information we gather, analyze, and share is accurate, comprehensible, and actionable. During an interview conducted for this book, ePatient Dave asserted, "No one can perform at their best potential if they don't have the right information." It is a mantra he shares often. His latest book is called *Let Patients Help* and also focuses on how patients can—and must—be a central part of the treatment process.

For a long time, it has been up to people like ePatient Dave to fight this battle. They navigate complex systems, demand access to their own data, and break new ground in patient empowerment. But, the odds have been stacked against them. Technology is not integrated. Medical collaboration is oftentimes minimal and inefficient. And perhaps most importantly, the ability to personalize care is too costly and complex.

Today, all of this is changing dramatically.

The fictional tales we used to begin the story of this book are meant to help you understand some of the ways mobile technology, genomics, sensors, and other new health tools are poised to benefit patients, caregivers, and physicians. In each story, we illustrated how technology-delivered health information can help people make more informed decisions, receive better quality care (and outcomes), and face the future with confidence rather than fear.

In Martha's case, you saw how the information she gathered via the diagnostic and knowledge tools available to her today left her worried and uncertain about her daughter's condition; however, by using a powerful sensing device, real-time data, and virtual medical advice, Martha was able to manage her daughter's fever appropriately.

In Henry's story, advances in genetics, electronic medical records, and mobile health applications helped him receive more personalized treatment options and guidance from his doctor. Virtual social tools also provided support from others who were dealing with a similar diagnosis, helping him manage his condition both emotionally and physically.

Today, we are witnessing the birth and evolution of a range of technologies, behaviors, and systems that will radically transform how we think about and manage health. Recognizing the overall shape and scope of the changes to come will require a big picture perspective on how these technologies will work together (and separately) to influence each of us in positive and negative ways. This will happen regardless of our background, proficiency with technology, temperament, and status (e.g., patient, caregiver, or observer).

The goal of this book is to share 15 trends that are poised to fundamentally change the way health and medical care is delivered and received in the near future. Rather than focus primarily on new technologies, our approach is decidedly human-centric. We look at how people will start to think and act differently in health, and position technology as an enabler for some of the changes to come.

As we outline these trends, we will share information about the process we used for identification and quantification, which included a combination of original research and curation, plus analysis of existing innovations and activities from pioneering medical systems and startups around the world. In the process, we uncovered the fact that these trends naturally aligned around several themes that are emerging because of three big challenges the health industry faces today:

- **Problem #1: Skyrocketing Medical Costs** - Thanks to the growing need for medical care, changes in legislative policy, and more costly treatment options—expenses related to medical care are dramatically increasing day by day.
- **Problem #2: Generic Medicine** - The standardized models that encourage universal treatment courses for patients are widely understood to be lacking; yet these approaches still dominate how medical care is delivered.
- **Problem #3: Limited Social Support** - Dealing with diseases or conditions (particularly when they are more rare) can be a solitary experience and support from outside the medical community from family, friends, and other patients can often be missing or lacking coordination.

Later in this book, we'll outline each of these problems in more detail, as well as the associated themes that describe how people have responded to these issues; however, first we'll briefly describe these themes below to provide you with additional context.

THEME #1 - HEALTH HYPEREFFICIENCY
Innovations in computing technologies are helping to make health and medical care more efficient, safe, and effective for all patients.

THEME #2 - THE PERSONALIZED HEALTH MOVEMENT
A philosophical and operational shift that considers the unique genetics, behaviors, and medical histories of individuals—instead of treating them based on inflexible or non-personalized guidelines and traditions.

THEME #3 - DIGITAL PEER-TO-PEER HEALTH CARE
A range of Web, social, and mobile tools are helping patients collaborate on things like navigating the new health insurance landscape, selecting providers, assisting in their own care, and providing emotional support.

What Are the 15 Trends?

Of course, describing the impact of technology on health at a macro level is only the first step. An outgrowth of the deep research and analysis conducted for this book was our identification of 15 unique trends that illustrate exactly how health care is changing on all levels.

Some trends are directly related to how patients experience care and the new and unique ways they are managing their treatment. Other trends illustrate the impact of technology on age-old medical traditions and practices. Below are the 15 trends (including the theme they fall under) and a short summary of each.

HEALTH HYPEREFFICIENCY
(How Technology and Computing Are Making Health Care
More Efficient, Safe, and Effective)

Trend #1 – Empathetic Interfaces: Health technology moves beyond focusing mainly on accuracy and functionality to incorporate more intuitive design and processes aimed at making digital tools more responsive to emotional needs, or more human-like.

Trend #2 – Unhealthy Surveillance: New surveillance technologies combine large amounts of digital, clinical, and behavioral data to track the health of individuals or groups and also raise significant privacy and security concerns.

Trend #3 – Predictive Psychohistory: Big Data, in combination with powerful computers, are increasingly being used to make large- and small-scale predictions about individual and population health.

THE PERSONALIZED HEALTH MOVEMENT
(How Technology is Helping Health Become More Individualized and Relevant to People's Needs)

Trend #4 – The Over-Quantified Self: As the volume of clinical and health information collected from wearable computers, passive sensors, and more increases, consumers will struggle to find true actionable value beyond "feel good stats" in this flood of data.

Trend #5 – Medical Genealogy: Genomics and advances in genealogy will combine to allow patients (and providers) to use ancestral history and genetics to predict the risk of disease, how they may respond to medications, and more. Over time, this valuable data may be passed on to future generations.

Trend #6 – Augmented Nutrition: A growing number of tools and technologies provides instant access to detailed nutritional information to help consumers make healthier choices in real-time about what to buy in stores or consume in restaurants.

Trend #7 – Healthy Real Estate: Increasing awareness of the role communities play in health and wellbeing will influence where people choose to rent or buy homes. Key considerations will include whether streets are walkable, the quality of nearby care, and access to social or religious institutions.

Trend #8 – The Device Divide: An outgrowth of the digital divide (disparities in access to digital technologies), financial considerations may prevent patients, providers, hospitals, and clinics from accessing the latest technological innovations in health.

Trend #9 – Multicultural Misalignment: Health technologies will be less effective if they are not optimized to account for differences in age, ethnicity, culture, and more. A range of organizations and businesses will work to provide unique and effective digital health tools to diverse populations.

Trend #10 – Natural Medicine: New science will continue to validate old beliefs about the value of spices, tonics, and herbs. This will result in more mainstream credibility for natural remedies that were once dismissively called "alternative medicine," but now have a body of tangible results to prove their value once and for all.

Trend #11 – MicroHealth Rewards: Inspired by federal legislation and a deeper understanding of behavioral science, insurers, corporations, health providers, and others will apply game theory to encourage people to adopt and sustain healthy behaviors by offering them tangible rewards (or punishments) as incentives.

Trend #12 – Neuro-Influence Mapping: Advances in brain imaging technology offer new insights into patients' behavioral profiles to support the development of unique personalized treatment programs that factor in which method of influence (fear, authority, conforming, etc.) may be most likely to work. These tools are also being used to shape marketing efforts in advertising and beyond.

DIGITAL PEER-TO-PEER HEALTH CARE
(How Digital Tools Are Enabling Enhanced
Collaboration and Peer Support)

Trend #13 – Virtual Counseling: Seeking emotional and logistical support, people forge one-to-one relationships online to offer assistance with navigating the new health insurance landscape, provide virtual moral support, "sponsor" one another, and share unique knowledge about conditions, ailments, and caregiving.

Trend #14 – CareHacking: Forced to increasingly take responsibility for their own care in a complex system, digitally savvy health consumers combine information from doctors, the Web, electronic medical records, and other sources to "hack" the health system in an effort to educate themselves, navigate loopholes, and ultimately get better, lower cost, and faster care for themselves and those they love.

Trend #15 – Accelerated Trial-Sourcing: Patients with chronic diseases and other conditions use digital tools to find one another, complete the usually costly and complex first stage of discovery for a clinical study, and then recruit the right pharmaceutical firms or other researchers to conduct the research.

In the next chapter we will outline our process for identifying the trends and share more on our method for quantifying and measuring each.

Much of this book will be devoted to detailing the trends—one per chapter. We'll also look at some of the fundamental forces shaping each trend. In addition, we will share original insights from the research we conducted in preparing this book. Finally, for each, we will share examples and case studies of how companies and entrepreneurs are already leveraging each trend to create new businesses, drive innovation, and improve health.

While we have written this book to be read in sequence, it is our assumption that some of you may skip to the trends you find particularly interesting or relevant. It's okay, we're not offended. Unlike a great piece of fiction, this book allows for flexibility and we encourage you to read it in the way that is most valuable to you.

Some Basic Definitions

Before continuing, we think it's important to spend a few moments defining a few critical health technology terms that are used throughout this book. (We'll define ePatients in the next chapter.) While many of you may be familiar with these terms, explaining them will help ensure clarity, including how we'll use them and why. You'll note that these terms are related and, because of this, we'll use them interchangeably throughout this book.

- **Digital Health:** The definition of this term is still evolving. Overall, it refers to how a range of technologies, including mobile, games, genetics, and social media are, according to Wikipedia, "empowering us to better track, manage, and improve our own and family's health." [1]
- **Health 2.0:** Like the term digital health, Health 2.0 refers to the use of mobile, electronic medical records, social media, and other technologies in health and wellness.
- **Health Technology:** We use the term health technology when referring to the use of digital tools such as social media, data analytics, mobile, and more to monitor, enhance, promote, and predict health.

In the next chapter, we talk about what makes an ePatient, our research and writing process, more on what this book is designed to achieve, and how it can help you.

The Background
How This Book Was Curated, and Why ePatients Matter

"We are the Gallery that walks. We are the Patients that wear our stories on our backs. Soon we shall come to a city near you and create gallery space in moments." — Regina Holliday, Patient Advocate and Artist [2]

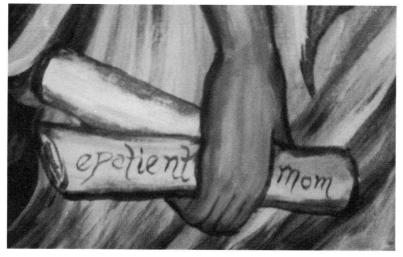

ePatient Mom, 2012 by Regina Holliday, Used With Permission

There is a quantifiable moment when people become ePatients. For some, it's during the process of being confronted with a difficult diagnosis and turning to the Internet for answers. For others, it's within the process of caring for a loved one who is struggling with a condition, and later dealing with the emptiness that comes after he or she passes away.

Regina Holliday is an artist and activist who well knows the world of ePatients. Forced to navigate the inefficient care system on behalf of her late husband Fred, she became a leading advocate in the movement for clarity and transparency in medical records after he passed away. Today she gives over 70 speeches a year at conferences and private summits. In many of those speeches, she shares the story of one of her most powerful projects: the "Walking Gallery."

Inspired by a single request to paint one of her murals on the back of a jacket of another ePatient, the Walking Gallery evolved as a collection of these jackets that visually tells various stories of patient empowerment. When someone wears one to an event, she describes the moment as one of disconnection. People stare at you. You enter the world of the "ostracized." And, for those who are not ePatients, it may be the closest experience to that of an actual patient traveling through a sometimes-heartless medical system.

Holliday started painting the jackets to offer a visible voice to the silently suffering. Her jackets are a symbol of that, but they also signify a greater movement, a movement where patients are no longer willing to silently suffer or blindly follow directions; instead, they are participating. They are making demands to control their destinies and data. They are empowered.

This empowerment is the fundamental emotion at the heart of this book, and has been well documented for some time now.

In November 2000, Susannah Fox and Lee Rainie of the Pew Research Center released the results of a first-of-its-kind survey examining how Americans were using the Web to seek health and medical information. Pew's report, *The Online Health Care Revolution: How the Web Helps Americans Take Better Care of Themselves*, helped to shed light on how the Internet had become a vital source of on-demand health information for many and was shaping people's medical decisions. [3]

While Pew's report helped to quantify the impact of the Web on Americans' health, they weren't the only ones to examine how patients could use the Internet for medical and wellness purposes. The late Tom Ferguson, MD, had long been a proponent of using digital resources to improve the doctor-patient relationship and helped to educate others on this topic. His book, *Health Online: How to Find Health Information, Support Groups, and Self-Help Communities in Cyberspace*, published in 1995 became a vital resource for people seeking informed guidance on how to use the Web to forge connections and find information. [4] Ferguson also coined the term ePatients, or "individuals who are equipped, enabled, empowered, and engaged in their health and health-care decisions."[5, 6]

Pew's report and Ferguson's book sparked a national conversation about the Web's role in patient education and empowerment and advanced our understanding of the ePatient revolution in other ways. Most importantly, the Robert Wood Johnson Foundation asked Ferguson to convene a research project designed to analyze how ePatients were influencing multiple aspects of the health system. In response, Ferguson convened a group of researchers, experts, and others into what became the ePatient Scholars Working Group.

In 2007, after Ferguson's untimely death from multiple myeloma, the Working Group published a groundbreaking white paper, e-Patients: *How They Can Help Us Heal Health Care*. [5] The paper, conceived and shaped by Ferguson, achieved several important milestones; it:

- Explored the growing ePatient movement
- Helped to put a human face to the ways people were using technology for health
- Charted how the Web was challenging and redefining many aspects of the patient-physician relationship

Since the ePatients white paper was published, the world has changed. The act of using the Web to find health information is no longer a novel concept. Mobile devices have helped to greatly expand Internet access (especially among African Americans and Hispanics) while making health information more accessible to people looking for support and education on the go. [7] We are about to enter an age where wearable devices such as watches and glasses, packed with sensors that can track heart rate, blood pressure, and other aspects of our health, will become the norm.

Are They Still ePatients?

In the midst of these profound technological changes, some have questioned whether it is still appropriate to use the term ePatient. [6] We believe it is. Just like in the early days of the Internet, we are beginning to see a new class of health consumers (patients, caregivers, and others), or ePatients, embrace novel technologies that:

- **Equip** them to monitor and analyze a range of sophisticated information about their health and wellbeing. For example, the Scanadu Scout, a new sensing device targeted toward the consumer market, measures pulse wave transit time (PWTT), or the "time it takes for a beat from [the] heart to reach somewhere else in [the] body." [8] PWTT can help determine the extent and severity of high blood pressure and is normally measured in the hospital, clinic, or other health institution.
- **Empower** them to take more control of the shape and scope of their care, from selecting procedures based on quality and cost, to using personal genetic information to understand whether a medication will be helpful or harmful before it is prescribed.
- **Engage** in their own wellbeing via technologies that provide them with constant feedback on how personal decisions (such as whether to eat a greasy hamburger or skip the gym) influence short- and long-term health.

How the ePatient Movement Evolved Beyond the Web

Traditionally, discussions about the ePatient movement have focused on how consumers are using the Internet to manage their care. For example, in 2007 Dr. Scott Haig wrote an infamous essay for *Time* relating the tale of "Susan," a patient he believed had been harmed by Dr. Google. Haig described her as full of "mispronounced words and half-baked ideas" she'd gotten from the Internet. [9] Haig's response to medical Googlers is similar to other physicians who feel threatened or frustrated by patients seeking to engage their doctors using sometimes inaccurate or incomplete information they gather from the Web.

Today, physicians and other health providers are far more comfortable interacting with Internet-using patients. [10] In fact, an increasing number of well-funded new organizations such as the Bucksbaum Institute are devoting themselves to fostering better doctor-patient communication. At the Institute, the focus is on helping medical students "preserve the sense of kindness . . . [before technology and process beats] it out of them." [11]

Yet, a host of technologies beyond the Web are poised to test the physician-patient relationship anew. What will happen, for instance, when patients begin to engage in conversations about whether a medication is safe and effective based on data gathered via genetic testing or a sensing device? Will physicians and other health-care providers react positively or negatively?

The time has come to expand our definition of ePatients beyond the Internet, and even mobile and social media, which have been major areas of focus over the past several years. [12] Instead, we need to consider how:

- Consumers will collect, share, and use information shaped by devices that allow them to continuously monitor their bodies
- Patients' treatment will be influenced by technologies they may know little about, but provide health-care providers and others with the power to predict and affect how they think and act in unanticipated ways
- ePatients' health data exhaust may benefit or harm them, this is especially important in an era where new organizations—many of them unfamiliar with health and medicine—begin collecting and analyzing vast amounts of medical information
- A new group of digitally savvy caregivers (taking care of their parents or others) will continue to grow
- The social connections patients forge through technology will influence how we conduct medical research, manage care, and more

Here's the bottom line: A more powerful, knowledgeable, and savvy ePatient is emerging. Our goal is to help you anticipate, understand, and perhaps even become this new ePatient—whether you work with (or for) one, care for one, or become one in the near or far future.

Why We Wrote This Book

Together, we (Rohit and Fard) possess close to three decades of experience working with patients, health-care professionals, insurance companies, hospitals, and others across the health system. During this time—especially in the last decade—we have seen a range of technological tsunamis strike the health industry, from the Internet to social media and now mobile. Each time, few in health have been prepared for the changes caused by these technologies. Most have been left scrambling to figure out how to navigate the new world they suddenly find themselves inhabiting. We believe avoiding "digital health shock" requires spending more time thinking ahead about the scope, implications, and role of technology.

Another phenomenon we've witnessed is the fact that conversations about health technologies are often divorced from the broad human and environmental (political, economic) factors that make them relevant and powerful. Fundamentally, we see five reasons for this gulf:

1. **Focus on Economics, Not Health Care:** Thanks to political and policymaking changes in the U.S. and elsewhere, there is global attention on not only the costs of health care, but how expenses can be contained and who should pay.
2. **Focus on Machines, Not Humans:** Sometimes we forget that people are at the center of health. Health and medical care is always going to be about how humans use digital tools to extend life, improve wellness, and accelerate happiness.
3. **Focus on Data, Not Motivations:** We tend to be much more interested in statistics about how many people are downloading mobile health applications rather than questions such as why we track our diet and exercise status using smartphones in the first place.
4. **Focus on Technology Trends, Not Health Industry Trends:** It's exciting to talk about how much venture capitalists have invested in certain startups and

new digital health tools; however, we'd have a better appreciation of why these firms and technologies are important if we were to examine the large-scale industry trends (e.g., increasing cost pressures, our aging population) contributing to their development and evolution.

5. **Focus on Digital Health Silos, Not Synergies:** In our multi-screen, multi-channel world, it has become clear that people are using many different technologies simultaneously for entertainment, education, and more. The same thing is happening in health as people use a combination of mobile applications, wearables like the Fitbit, and more to monitor and manage their health. Despite this, we don't spend enough time thinking about how a variety of digital health tools are (or can) be used together to educate, inform or change how people behave.

It is this missing conversation we want to help drive—by making a deeper connection between the effects of technology in health care and the fundamental changes in how patients, caregivers, and others think about, act on, and are informed about health.

Who Should Read This Book?

Given the intense interest in digital health, we know many different people may read this book. In particular, here are a few audiences we expect may find value in this publication, including some details on what each should expect to learn:

- **Patients and Caregivers:** Possess a road map that can be used to understand the technological resources that will become widely available, the forces shaping medical care, and people's motivations for selecting and using certain digital tools for health
- **Entrepreneurs:** Understand the broad forces shaping how ePatients are using digital tools to navigate health in order to develop better products and services
- **Physicians and Other Health-Care Providers:** Recognize how ePatients will soon have access to a broader array of health information sources beyond the Web; some of the information people will start bringing to doctors will be more personalized and enhanced by in-depth medical data
- **Health Executives (from Pharmaceutical Companies, Insurance Firms,**

Hospitals, etc.): Appreciate how technology will empower consumers to make more informed choices about the treatments and drugs they select

- **Health Communicators and Marketers:** Be informed about consumer activities, motivations for selecting and using digital health technologies, and broad industry trends that will influence how people are informed about health and wellness

Overall, our focus on big picture issues in health shaped our analysis of the 15 ePatient trends (lightly or heavily influenced by digital technologies) we outline in this book. In some cases, we examine emerging movements such as health self-tracking (quantified self), or the act of monitoring health indicators such as blood pressure and heart rate, and ask if there is a dark side to these trends. In others, we look at what it will mean if we have powerful computer programs that can collect and analyze vast amounts of health data in order to make predictions about people's individual future health.

Our discussion about these trends will feature not only quantifiable research and analysis of the positives and negatives, but will also highlight tangible examples of how they are playing out through real-life stories and examples.

How Did We Identify the Trends Outlined in This Book?

In previous books such as *Likeonomics* as well as his popular annual Trend Report, Rohit described his research process as being heavily focused on curation, multiple conversations with visionary people, and being informed by his work with some of the largest brands in the world. Fard's insights are influenced by the in-depth research he has conducted with health consumers for nearly a decade, experience defining and describing the digital health future for large and small health organizations globally, and work with a variety of health and wellness brands.

For this collaboration, we have combined our research styles to identify and explore the trends described in this book in four important ways:

1. **Filtering Signal from Noise:** We have collected and analyzed dozens of individual digital health trends, from augmented reality to wearable computing, and filtered them according to a single criterion: How will these tools and technologies work together to help ePatients achieve specific goals related to their health and wellbeing?

2. **Conducting Original Research With ePatients:** In late 2012, Fard's firm Enspektos launched a unique research project called digihealth pulse. One goal of this study is to uncover new information on how digitally active ePatients (those who turn to the Web and social media regularly and also have used the Internet to search for health information) view and use a range of emerging digital health technologies. Another objective is to look at how ePatients react to digital health content when they are being passively observed using the Web and social media. A range of data from digihealth pulse (most of it collected by Enspektos in late 2013 specifically for this book) is provided throughout this publication. See Appendix I for more information about digihealth pulse.

3. **Picking Experts' Brains:** In addition to curation and original research, we conducted interviews with patients, entrepreneurs, and others. We are grateful for their participation, as they helped us to further understand the scope and implications of these trends.

4. **Analysis of Funding Activity:** We also looked at recent professional and consumer investment activity in the digital health space. Since 2012, health technology funding has increased, especially for products and services targeted toward consumers, tools that enable remote patient-provider interaction, and devices that help people track their health status. [13, 14]

As you have learned, ePatients are not only still relevant, but beginning to use a range of technologies and tools that are providing them with greater insight and information about their health. In the next chapter, we take a step back to examine key big picture problems, patterns, and more that are helping to drive the evolving ePatient movement.

The Big Picture:
How Three Big Themes Describe All of the Trends in This Book

Humans are notoriously bad at anticipating change. And once change happens, getting large groups of people to react and adapt to it is an even tougher challenge. In response, those who have the privilege (and burden) of leading change will try almost anything to make the process work just a little bit faster.

Expert communicators and politicians will use powerful stories to tap into and ignite our emotions. Economists will try to motivate and predict behavior change by applying various incentive and reward models. And, change management consultants will turn to one of their favorite methods: stories about frogs.

Actually, one frog story in particular gets more than its fair share of mentions. Perhaps you've heard it before . . .

If you place a frog into a pot of boiling water, it will jump out. If you put it in a pot of cold water and slowly heat it, the frog won't react and will boil to death.

This story has become the ultimate anecdote to explain the dangers of complacency and why change is essential. There's only one problem with this tale of slowly boiling frogs: it isn't true.

Back in 1995, *Fast Company's* (unfortunately) fictional "Consultant Debunking Unit" took a closer look at the boiling frog story. [15] The magazine asked a question that would occur to any good scientist: What would a frog actually do in this situation? To find out, *Fast Company* shared this story with Dr. George R. Zug, a longtime curator of reptiles and amphibians at the National Museum of Natural History, and asked him to rate its accuracy. Zug replied: "Well that's, may I say, bullshit. If a frog had a means of getting out, it certainly would get out." [15]

In addition to seeking colorful expert commentary, *Fast Company* conducted its own experiment. Perhaps deciding against immediately killing an innocent frog by placing it into a pot of boiling water, magazine staffers tested how long it would take two frogs to react to being placed in slowly warming liquid. "We [put] Frog A into a pot of cold water and applied moderate heat. At 4.20 seconds, it safely exited the pot with a leap of 24 centimeters. We then placed Frog B into a pot of lukewarm water and applied moderate heat. At 1.57 seconds, it safely exited the pot with a leap of 57 centimeters." [15]

We share this tale of the "underestimated frog" to underscore an important point about the philosophy and approach behind this book. We know that stories can be helpful to illustrate ideas, but they lose credibility without the right foundation in facts and research. Throughout this chapter (and book), we will also share stories to bring our ideas to life, but whenever we do, you can be sure that they are backed up with plenty of evidence.

So, let's get started by turning our lens towards three critical problems facing the health industry today and the major shifts these issues have inspired.

3 Major Problems and Shifts in Health

The quest to solve several major health system problems has contributed to the rise of three digital health themes that describe how ePatients use technology, receive treatment, are informed about health, and more. These problems, and their associated themes, are illustrated in Figure I and described below.

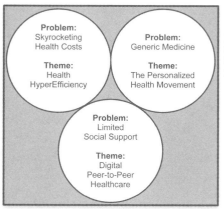

Figure I:
Significant Problems
Contributing to the Rise of
Major Health Technology Themes

Problem #1: Skyrocketing Health Costs

Many discussions about the high cost of health care begin by citing the trillions of dollars, euros, pounds, and other currencies spent each year on medical procedures, prescription medications, and more. While these statistics may be shocking, they are too abstract for most people to comprehend. We're going to bring things down to earth by focusing the cost discussion on two common stages of life that many can relate to: having a baby and getting older.

In June 2013, the *New York Times* published the second in a yearlong series of articles focusing on skyrocketing health expenses in the U.S. [16] Elisabeth Rosenthal, the author of the series, focused on what it costs to have a baby, especially for people whose insurance plans do not cover maternity care. When Renée Martin (who Rosenthal profiled in the article) asked her hospital to estimate the cost of her maternity care, she was given a very wide range of fees, between $4,000 and $45,000.

One reason for this wide disparity in costs is the fact that hospitals charge different rates to patients, health insurance companies, and government. It has become common for hospitals to send patients invoices and billing statements showing the list prices associated with various medical services; however, insurance firms and government don't pay retail. Doctors, hospitals, and others are reimbursed based on a much lower negotiated rate. On the other hand, uninsured or underinsured patients like Martin pay much higher rates, mainly because they do not have the power to negotiate lower fees.

Although large, so-called third party payers like insurance firms and government pay lower rates, they are also experiencing sticker shock from childbirth costs. According to an analysis published by Truven Health Analytics in 2013, expenses associated with maternal care increased by over 40% between 2004 and 2010 for women with private insurance. In addition, Medicaid paid on average, $4,000 more for babies born by C-section versus newborns delivered vaginally. [17] In fact, it costs more to have a baby in the United States than anywhere else in the world. [16]

Childbirth is but one area where rising health-care costs are a concern. As the U.S. population ages, some experts anticipate spending to increase significantly, partly because seniors are living longer with chronic diseases like diabetes and high blood pressure. [18] For example, Dr. Rhonda Randall, chief medical officer of UnitedHealthcare Medicare & Retirement, told USA Today in May 2013, "As generations move into retirement, they become greater consumers of health care. But those turning 65 today 'are more likely to live longer than their parents and grandparents, and much more likely to live sicker for a longer period of time.'" [18]

Also, while medical spending is higher for older Americans overall, it skyrockets at the end of seniors' lives. [19] According to the authors of a 2010 report published by the National Bureau of Economic Research, out-of-pocket costs associated with medical care "represent a numerically large and potentially important drain on financial resources, particularly for households as time of death nears." This may have an influence on how elderly people may spend their earnings as they "continue to hold (or even accumulate) wealth as a hedge against uninsured costs surrounding expensive end-of-life care-giving for themselves or their spouse." [19]

The good news is that innovations in health care are being developed that may enable us to more successfully tackle the cost problem, which explains our first big theme . . . Health HyperEfficiency.

WHAT IS HEALTH HYPEREFFICIENCY?
Innovations in computing technologies are helping to make health
and medical care more efficient, safe, and effective for all patients.

Inside the Impact of Health HyperEfficiency

While there are many factors contributing to the rise in health spending, the
examples of childbirth and aging outlined above help us focus on two, as they are
very relevant to our discussion:

- **Increased Demand for Health Services:** An aging population will always require more medical resources. Added to this, we are seeing younger people
  require more health care due to conditions such as childhood obesity and early
  onset of many preventable conditions such as type II diabetes and high blood
  pressure.
- **Limited Price Transparency:** With little information on the true costs of
  health care (and significant differences in what health institutions charge for
  the same procedures), it is difficult for consumers and others to limit spending
  or shop for high quality, less expensive treatment.

Over the years, businesses, legislators, consumers, and others have used a range of
tactics to reduce medical spending; however some, such as limiting (or rationing)
treatment, or releasing data on health costs (such as what hospitals charge the
government) remain controversial.

Some see a possible answer to the problem of skyrocketing costs in digital health
innovations. The potential value of digital technologies is twofold:

1. **Reduce the Demand for Health Services:** When technology is used in smart
   ways to track people's health, it can also be leveraged to make predictions
   about who may likely need care in the near and far future and offer data to
   help prevent sickness and death. In addition, the devices we use (mobile, etc.)
   can help to deliver more responsive, human-like experiences that do a better
   job of educating people on their health, helping them make better decisions,

and avoid costly medical care.

2. **Help People Select Cost-Effective and High Quality Care:** Digital technologies can automatically mine a range of health data on the quality of care, the cost of medical procedures, medications, and other factors. This information may be delivered to consumers, hospitals, insurance firms, businesses, and others to help them choose health products and services that are both cost-effective and high quality.

We refer to the group of digital tools offering these benefits and thereby helping to reduce health costs as *hyper-efficient* technologies[1]. In contrast to traditional tech, hyper-efficient tools can be used alone or in combination to:

- Collect and analyze large and diverse data sets (e.g., images, video, text, medical data, and more) faster and more accurately
- Make predictions about human behavior such as whether someone will become sick in the near future
- Enable people to engage with computers in ways that resemble how humans communicate with each other

In our discussion of future ePatient trends related to the Health HyperEfficiency movement, we will reference a range of technologies, which are described in Table I.

Table I: Technologies That Make Health HyperEfficiency Possible

Overview: Key Hyper-Efficiency Related Digital Technologies
Big Data: Over the past decade, the volume and types of data we are gathering about our bodies, the environment, digital activities (e.g., Web surfing), and more has vastly increased. The term Big Data traditionally refers to large and diverse data sets that are being generated and collected more quickly each year. It is also used in the context of tools, techniques, and technologies used to accurately analyze this information. [20] In health, Big Data is being used for a range of purposes, including helping doctors diagnose disease more accurately and delivering highly relevant and personalized health information to people.

Predictive Analytics: We are collecting large amounts of information about people's perceptions and past behaviors (e.g., the Web sites they visit, what they buy, who they vote for, their digital social connections, and more). This data can be analyzed to find patterns and correlations that suggest how people may think and act in the future. The art and science of predicting future actions using data is called predictive analytics. [21]

Health Surveillance and Sensing Technologies: A range of companies are producing technologies that allow us to monitor and measure our bodies in real-time, including Scanadu and Jawbone. These sensing devices are collecting information on many aspects of our health, including blood pressure, blood sugar, heart rate, cholesterol levels, and even whether we are taking medications as prescribed. From a surveillance perspective, monitoring and mining digital health content for insights has become a major business activity, especially within the pharmaceutical industry. [22]

Social Media and Social Networks: The rapid growth of social tools has enabled patient collaboration on an unprecedented level, which is allowing for everything from shared reviews of medical providers to patients sharing highly tactical advice on how to navigate the inefficiencies of the health care system.

Artificial Intelligence: Computing and programming power has advanced to the point where we can develop machines (from robots to mobile devices) that act in more human and responsive ways. Making computers more like people is what those advancing the field of artificial intelligence are working to achieve.

Problem #2: Generic Medicine

Over the past century or so, American health care has undergone many changes, especially in the area of personalized medicine; however, this meant something entirely different in the late 19th century. During that period, personalization referred to the fact that U.S. physicians would tailor their treatment strategies according to the needs (and whims) of individual patients, in contrast to their European counterparts. [23]

For example, the practice of medicine was heavily influenced by folk traditions, regional customs, and the use of cures passed down over many generations. In addition, almost any man of European ancestry could set up shop in a community and call himself a doctor. Because doctors relied on their clients for income and many were misinformed about the true causes of disease, medical care was both highly personalized and varied depending on the region, or even the person delivering care. [23] In many respects, personal relationships rather than medical knowledge or skill determined the fate of physicians practicing during this period. [23]

Over time, especially in the beginning of the 20th century, medical care became significantly less tailored toward the individual and based on standard scientific principles. By the 1920s, physicians were required to be licensed to practice medicine and using "natural" or homeopathic remedies fell out of favor among medical professionals. [24]

Standardization resulted in many benefits, including making medicine safer and more effective. This was mainly due to the fact that many patients began to be treated using a range of standardized criteria developed based on what came to be known as evidence-based medicine; however, standardization also had negative consequences. [25] For example, prior to recent times, much of the research used to shape treatment strategies was limited or flawed because it was based on medical studies that were conducted primarily with white men and excluded or under-represented women, ethnic and racial minorities, people with rare conditions, and others. [26] This is important because over time researchers have learned that certain medications are more or less effective due to a number of factors such as:

- **Patients' Backgrounds:** Some drugs are absorbed or processed differently by people of various ethnic and racial backgrounds [27]
- **Personal Genetic Factors:** Certain medications work differently depending on specific genetic characteristics shared by groups of people [28]

Another drawback of standardization and changes in the structure and financing of medicine is that patients have steadily received less personal attention from physicians over time. For example, a study cited by the *New York Times* in 2013 revealed that new physicians spend an average of just eight minutes speaking face-to-face with patients. [29]

The combination of lack of personalized attention from physicians and the limitations of medical research have contributed to a problem we call generic medicine. Note that we are not referring to the use of generic medications here, but rather to the misguided beliefs (below) which have led directly to the rise in generic medicine:

- **One-size-fits-all health management strategies** that do not account for preferences, genetics, environment, family situations, or other personal factors
- **Limited price transparency and tools** that enable patients to select providers and care, based on cost and quality factors
- **Dismissal of alternative or non-Western medical practices** based on a lack of knowledge about research examining whether these treatments are safe and effective
- **Failure to deliver health content and incentives** that are relevant and meaningful for individuals rather than broad groups

The good news is the medical community is moving away from generic medicine, which explains our second big theme . . . The Personalized Health Movement.

WHAT IS THE PERSONALIZED HEALTH MOVEMENT?

A philosophical and operational shift that considers the unique genetics, behaviors, and medical histories of individuals instead of treating them based on inflexible or non-personalized guidelines and traditions.

Inside the Impact of the Personalized Health Movement

Generic medicine has been ascendant for many decades, but there are signs of hope that this approach to health care may be starting to wane. In 2011, the members of a Kauffman Foundation-funded research group published an extensive paper, *The Personalized Health Project*, documenting the evolution of the personalized health movement. [30] They defined personalized health as including "predictive tests and technologies for individuals and for society, and also science-based strategies to prevent or mitigate disease and poor health." Interestingly, they characterized personalized medicine, as a "subset of personalized health" referring to it as "therapies that can be tailored to an individual's own genetics and physiology."

The authors of the Kauffman-funded report included the rise of the patient consumer within the broader personalized health movement. Not only are patients using a range of social tools to connect, but they are also shaping the future direction of medical research. For example, PatientsLikeMe has conducted a number of patient-centered studies examining the safety and effectiveness of medications and various treatment strategies. [31]

The personal health movement is still evolving. Despite this, a growing number of patients, researchers, medical professionals, and others are investigating, developing, and implementing personalized health tools, techniques, and strategies that are outlined in Table II. We will discuss these further when describing ePatient trends related to the personalized health movement.

Table II: Technologies Associated With the Personalized Health Movement

Overview: Key Digital Technologies and Tools Powering the Personalized Health Movement
Genetic Profiling and Testing: In his book, *The Creative Destruction of Medicine*, Dr. Eric Topol outlines the pros, cons, and history of personal genomics, from the genetic tests offered by companies like 23andMe, to ongoing efforts to improve medication effectiveness by administering drugs based on patients' genetic profiles. [32] Today—especially as the cost of genetic testing decreases—more Americans are purchasing genetic tests for themselves and their families designed to help them understand their risk of disease.
The Internet, Mobile, and Wearable Health Devices: First widely introduced in 2003 by Stanford Professor B.J. Fogg, the theory of captology, or why human-computer interaction can help influence behavior, helped to increase understanding of how computing devices can be used to shape health and wellness. [33] Partly because of Fogg's work, we have a better understanding of how computers, mobile devices, the Web, and other tools can be used to deliver highly personalized health experiences designed to inform and persuade. The Internet and other technologies have become essential parts of many people's health and wellness experiences.
Ubiquitous Sensors: In her wide-ranging report, *Making Sense of Sensors: How New Technologies Can Change Patient Care*, Jane Sarasohn-Kahn outlined a future in which devices, or sensors that automatically collect a range of health data internally and externally, can help patients and doctors monitor health.[2] [34] Since Sarasohn-Kahn's report appeared in February 2013, sensors have attracted significant attention, as suggested by recent investment activity. If utilized appropriately, sensors may become a vital component of efforts to use personal health data to provide individualized care, prevent disease, and more.

Augmented Reality: Wikipedia characterizes augmented reality as the use of "computer-generated sensory input such as sound, video, graphics" or other data to enhance real world imagery. [35] For example, virtual information can be incorporated onto a photo of a famous landmark, including when it was built and the materials used to construct it. In health, augmented reality can be used for a number of tasks, including providing safety tips on how to properly use children's over-the-counter medicines when the product is viewed via a mobile device. Augmented reality can also help people make better food choices, such as providing nutritional information on top of an image showing a popular fast food item.

Brain Mapping: For centuries, the brain was the ultimate black box. We knew that information went in based on what we saw, tasted, touched, and felt, but little about what sensory input does to the brain. Today, neuroscientists have developed tools, such as functional magnetic resonance imaging and electroencephalograms that help us map conscious and unconscious responses to internal and external stimuli. Psychologists aren't the only ones using these tools. Marketers have been employing brain-scanning technologies to map and predict the influence of advertising and more. [36] Later, we'll also describe how neuroscience is being used to personalize health care, including in the area of mental health and addiction treatment.

Social Media: Social media tools, such as blogs, Facebook, and Twitter have steadily become more important to people seeking health and medical information. In fact, according to a Kantar Media study released in 2013, consumer use of social media sites for health research has increased by 21 percent since 2011. [37] Social content—especially if it is generated based on personal data, preferences, and requests—can aid in the delivery of individualized health information and care.

Problem #3: Limited Social Support

For years the social side of treatment and recovery remained underappreciated. The severe impact of debilitating mental conditions such as depression were minimized; emotional suffering was never given the same level of concern by the medical community as physical pain and suffering. This is all changing, and nowhere is it more apparent than in the world of caregiving.

Amy Goyer has worked in the field of aging for more than 30 years, but in many ways she was completely unprepared for the immense challenges she would face when she decided to become the primary caregiver for her two aging parents. Goyer, who serves as AARP's home and family expert, is often featured in the media speaking candidly about her caregiving experiences. One topic she frequently discusses is the social isolation she feels as she juggles caring for her parents and maintaining a career.

How does she cope? Goyer says she relies on digital tools such as the Web and social media to stay connected with others and receive support. In an August 2013 post published on the AARP blog, she related how e-mail helped her get through a particularly tough moment. She wrote: "Eight months after I'd relocated to Phoenix to help my parents, I found myself frozen, unable to drag myself out of bed and face my to-do list . . . I leaned out of bed far enough to reach my laptop and e-mailed some friends. Dorothy e-mailed back, "Do not succumb to the bed!!!" Her message made me laugh in spite of myself . . ." [38]

We recognize that many people coping with health issues have a hard time finding and receiving emotional and social support; however, we're highlighting caregivers because they face a unique burden. Caregivers must figure out how to take care of their loved ones and maintain their own wellbeing with limited resources. Lack of knowledge about the educational and social tools available to them provided by organizations such as AARP compounds the problems they face.

Over the coming years, many more Americans will face the challenges associated with caregiving, including social and emotional isolation. According to the Pew Research Center, thirty percent of U.S. adults defined themselves as caregivers in 2010. [39] In 2013, Pew reported that the caregiver population had increased by nine percent. [40] The number of caregivers is expected to continue increasing as the population gets older and age-related illnesses like dementia become more prevalent. [41]

The good news is that increasing numbers of caregivers are no longer facing this burden alone, which explains our third and final theme . . . Digital Peer-to-Peer Health Care.

WHAT IS DIGITAL PEER-TO-PEER HEALTH CARE?
A range of Web, social, and mobile tools are helping patients collaborate on things like navigating the new health insurance landscape, selecting providers, assisting in their own care, and providing emotional support.

Inside the Impact of Digital Peer-to-Peer Health Care

Ask Susannah Fox of the Pew Research Center, and a self-described "Internet Geologist" about the digital innovation that excites her most and she'll tell you it's "people talking with each other." [42] Communicating via e-mail, the Web, and social media (or simply face-to-face) may not be as sexy as Big Data or body sensing technologies, but Fox believes it's going to have a bigger impact on health.

In a 2013 post published on her personal blog, Fox explains why: "[T]echnology allows us to widen the network of people we can talk with, increase the velocity of these conversations, inject them with more source material, then archive and make them searchable." [42]

The Pew Research Center defines the phenomenon of digital technologies helping to forge connections between people as "peer-to-peer health care." [43] We've tweaked Pew's language slightly by defining this health trend as *digital peer-to-peer health care*, as our focus is on how tools like the Web and social media can help reduce patients' and caregivers' social isolation while improving their emotional wellbeing. In Table III we describe some of the technologies driving digital peer-to-peer health care.

Will digital peer-to-peer health care change the world? *It may already have.* Because of the Internet, countless patients, caregivers, and others have forged life-long connections that have benefited their physical and mental health. Medical data shared by patients is helping to transform long-standing beliefs about how we test medications and whether they are truly effective in the real world. And, from an individual perspective, Amy Goyer is testament to the fact that digital technologies have become integral to health, partly because of the bonds they help us form and maintain.

Table III: Technologies Powering Digital Peer-to-Peer Health Care

Overview: Key Digital Technologies and Tools Driving Peer-to-Peer Health Care
The Internet and Social Media: Over the past decade, the Web has become a significant source of social and emotional support for caregivers and patients, especially those with chronic conditions. Pew reports that caregivers are "heavy technology users," and highly likely to go online to gather health information and use the Web (and face-to-face conversations) to seek advice and support. [40] As for people with chronic diseases such as cancer and diabetes, while lower numbers possess Internet access, they are more likely to use it to search for health content and frequent social networks and other sites. [44]
Open Patient Networks: A growing number of patient-oriented networks are becoming *de-facto* trusted sources of information on particular disease conditions, displacing even authoritative peer-reviewed content that may be available online. These real-life melting pots of patient experience, such as PatientsLikeMe, are enabling anyone to share their stories within an established community, no matter where they happen to be in the world.
Mobile Health Applications: As mobile has become more popular in health, a number of organizations are developing mobile applications targeted toward patients and caregivers. For example, in July 2013, the U.S. Department of Veterans Affairs launched a pilot project in which it provided 1,000 iPads to veterans' caregivers pre-loaded with 10 customized applications. [45] There are thousands of medical mobile apps designed to help patients manage their care and U.S. federal regulators are taking steps to guide their development and even allow doctors to prescribe them. [46]

A Health-Care Theme Recap

In this chapter, we outlined three health-care themes that are emerging as people try to solve a number of major problems faced by patients, providers, caregivers, and others. As a short recap, here are the problems as well as the themes.

Problem: Skyrocketing Health Costs	Solution – Health HyperEfficiency: Innovations in computing technologies are helping to make health and medical care more efficient, safe, and effective for all patients.

Problem: Generic Medicine	Solution – The Personalized Health Movement: A philosophical and operational shift that considers the unique genetics, behaviors, and medical histories of individuals instead of treating them based on inflexible or non-personalized guidelines and traditions.
Problem: Limited Social Support	Solution – Digital Peer-to-Peer Health Care: A range of Web, social, and mobile tools are helping patients collaborate on things like navigating the new health insurance landscape, selecting providers, assisting in their own care, and providing emotional support.

Now that we have outlined major health industry issues influencing the evolution and use of technology, let's turn our focus to discussing the unique ways ePatients are being impacted by these themes. After pausing for a brief interlude, we'll begin our analysis in Part I, starting with Health HyperEfficiency.

---

[1] While our primary focus has been on how these tools can be used to reduce spending, we will discuss other use cases throughout this book.

[2] While sensors that allow patients and providers to monitor health externally are well known, a new class of devices that can be embedded into prescription medicines, such as one developed by Proteus Digital Health, are gaining increased attention.

Interlude:
How the Trends Are Organized and Described

The rest of this book will take you on a journey inside the 15 major trends in health care that are changing the ways consumers (patients, caregivers) receive treatment, consume information, and support one another.

Each of these 15 trends represents technologies and issues that our research and analysis indicates will become increasingly important between now and 2015 (as well as beyond).

For each trend, we will provide context to help you understand why it is important and examples of how this trend is taking shape today. In particular, we will use the following format to describe each trend:

- **Organizational Framework:** The 15 trends are grouped based on the themes (Health HyperEfficiency, Digital Peer-to-Peer Health Care, the Personalized Health Movement) described previously (see Figure II).
- **Trend Summary:** We summarize each trend and provide additional background information on its history, scope, and importance.
- **digihealth pulse ePatient Data Analysis:** For certain trends, we feature data collected via Enspektos' digihealth pulse research initiative (see Appendix I for more information about digihealth pulse).
- **Stories:** For most trends, we provide examples of companies and other organizations either helping to advance these trends, or solving problems associated

with them.

As you review these trends you'll note that we've also highlighted some of the negative consequences of health technologies. Some may hesitate to examine digital health's shortcomings, but we feel doing so is vitally important if we are to fully appreciate its impact.

We will also offer insights on how and why these trends matter, both from the perspective of engaged patients, and others who are part of the health industry.

Figure II: Emerging ePatient Trends Related to the Themes Introduced Previously

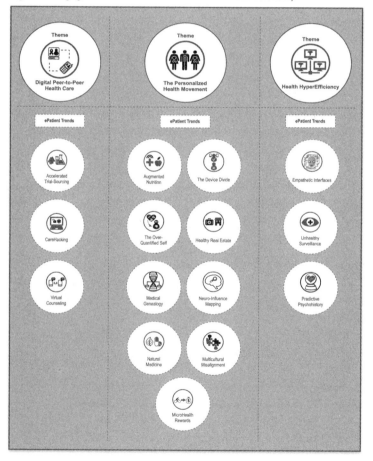

After you absorb these trends, some of you may be looking for advice on what to do about them. For example, how should people protect sensitive health data or prevent information overload? We do offer some high-level guidance in the final chapter on these questions; however, the answers heavily depend on what audience category you happen to fall into. As a result, we don't focus as much on tactical advice in each trend, but rather on providing you with the context and research behind it so that you can begin to develop your own plan of action for how to utilize the information we provide independently.

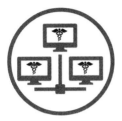

Part 1:
Health HyperEfficiency:
From Human-Like Computer Interfaces to Data-Powered Oracles

"We now are entering the Cognitive Systems Era, in which a new generation of computing systems is emerging with embedded data analytics, automated management and data-centric architectures . . ."

- Dr. Martin Kohn, Chief Medical Scientist, IBM Research [47]

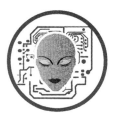

Trend 1:
Empathetic Interfaces

Artificial intelligence, improved user interfaces, and wearable devices are coming together to make health technology go beyond the diagnostic to be more empathetic and responsive to emotional needs—in other words . . . more human.

Hiroshi Ishiguro has found the ultimate way to avoid attending meetings. A renowned Japanese engineer, Ishiguro received worldwide attention when he developed an android replica of himself so lifelike that he could regularly operate it remotely and send it to meetings on his behalf. [48]

On a day when Ishiguro may have been continuing his efforts to test the boundaries of human-android interaction, a group of Japanese school children were peppering an unexpected source with questions. "Where's the bathroom?" one child asked. Calm and smiling, she turned toward the child and replied, "The bathroom is located east of here." "You are wise," another child yells. "No way! You are wiser than me," she responds.

Ordinarily, this conversation would not be worth noting, but there's something very special about it. The children were asking questions of a human-like android, Actroid-SIT, which was developed by the Japanese robotics firm Kokoro. Actroid-SIT is special because Kokoro has made a number of modifications to the android in an attempt to make it more empathetic and responsive to people. According to a 2013 report published in *IEEE Spectrum*, researchers tweaked the robot's programming so that it would change subjects when interrupted and point, wave, and look directly at people speaking with it. [49]

These minor modifications had a significant impact on people's perceptions of the robot. *IEEE Spectrum* reported those interacting with Actroid-SIT "called the android more friendly, sophisticated, and warm when the new gesturing system was used, compared to the normal gesturing approach." [49]

Most experts agree that we are years away from the point where we will see lifelike androids—either operated by people or powered by artificial intelligence—roaming the streets (although it is likely this will happen in Japan first); however, the concept of making computer-human interfaces more empathetic is gaining ground in a range of industries, including health. Below, we discuss two critical areas where empathetic interfaces are currently making a difference: preventing people from re-entering the hospital after they are discharged and improving employee health.

Reducing Hospital Readmissions and Powering Corporate Wellness Initiatives With Empathetic Interfaces

In recent years, much of the public conversation and controversy related to the U.S. legislation, the Affordable Care Act (better known as Obamacare), has focused on penalties individuals and businesses must pay for not providing or securing health insurance coverage; however, there are other parts of the law that have received less attention but have already had significant impact on medical care. One of these is the Hospital Readmissions Reduction Program, which is described in Section 3025 of the Act. [50]

Overall, the program is designed to reduce Medicare costs associated with patients who enter the hospital, but are shortly readmitted, usually within less than 30 days. In 2012, the *New York Times* reported that "one in five Medicare patients returns to the hospital within a month . . . readmissions cost the government more than $17 billion annually." [51] The Centers for Medicare and Medicaid Services (CMS) issued a rule (in 2012) requiring hospitals to pay penalties for Medicare patients who reenter the hospital within 30 days of being discharged across a range of conditions, beginning with heart attack, heart failure, and pneumonia. [52]

Uncertainty about whether the Affordable Care Act would survive a Supreme Court challenge and concerns about how the government would measure readmission rates (especially among hospitals serving the poor) gave some executives the impression that the penalties might be avoided or reduced. [53] Yet, right on schedule, CMS announced that it had fined 2,217 hospitals a total of $280 million for high readmission rates in 2012. [54] A year later, CMS cited 2,225 hospitals for elevated re-hospitalization rates for a total of $227 million. [55]

Some health insurance companies are following the federal government's lead when it comes to launching new initiatives to reduce costs associated with hospital readmissions. For example, in July 2012, Highmark announced that it would begin paying hospitals between 1 and 3 percent less if they did not meet its standards for preventing the readmission of patients fewer than 30 days after they were discharged from the hospital. [56] Highmark's effort focused on hospitals participating in its pay-for-performance program, which rewards hospitals for meeting certain health quality targets such as cancer screenings or the number of people maintaining healthy cholesterol levels.

Nurses, physicians, home health-care providers, and others generally serve at the front lines of efforts to reduce readmissions; however, until recently, they have not received the human or technological support they need to follow up with patients outside the hospital to reduce readmissions. Recent public and private sector efforts to reduce readmission-related costs have changed this dynamic. Now, insurers, hospitals, and others are starting to use (and give health-care providers access to) a range of technologies—some featuring empathetic interfaces—to solve the readmission problem.

Two readmission prevention tools include remote patient monitoring and predictive analytics. Remote patient monitoring refers to the use of sensing devices to monitor patients' wellbeing. This can involve utilizing technologies that measure whether how well patients with heart failure or who had a heart attack are performing at home after they leave the hospital. Predictive analytics (or the science of using data to predict the future) can be used to anticipate which patients are at the highest risk of being readmitted to the hospital. For example, in 2013 the College of Healthcare Information Management Executives published a case study focusing on how California's El Camino Hospital used predictive analytics to reduce readmissions by 25 percent. [57]

El Camino Hospital didn't just rely on predictive analytics to reduce readmissions. It also employed telepresence, a remote monitoring technology that uses empathetic interfaces (such as two-way video) to connect patients and health providers inside and outside the hospital. [58]

Another telepresence solution currently undergoing testing is remotely operated health devices designed for in-home use. For example, the European Union is currently funding the development of the GiraffPlus program. The project gets its name from Giraff, a telepresence robot packed with a range of empathetic interfaces, including a video chatting interface that allows health providers, caregivers, and others to visit elderly patients at home. Giraff and a combination of sensing devices that can monitor blood pressure or detect a fall are being tested in Spain, Italy, and Sweden to determine whether GiraffPlus improves health. [59]

Can Human-Like Computer Coaches Boost Engagement in Corporate Wellness Programs?

Some employers offer employees programs designed to help them lose weight, quit smoking, exercise more, and eat healthier. Why? Most want happy and healthy workforces; however, money is another major reason organizations develop and promote wellness initiatives. It is estimated that employees who have chronic conditions like heart disease or are obese generate more than one-quarter of employers' health-care costs. [60]

This is part of the reason why some consider the workplace the first line of defense against a range of preventable health conditions. If employers can encourage employees to engage in healthier behaviors, we may avoid many diseases and reduce future medical expenses. This is the thinking behind another important, but widely under-reported feature of the Affordable Care Act: support for workplace wellness programs. For example, beginning in 2014, the federal government will allow employers to reward employees up to 30 percent of the total cost of their insurance premium for meeting specific health goals (e.g. losing weight or quitting smoking). [61, 62]

Given the current and future focus on workplace wellness initiatives, it makes sense to ask whether these programs work — and, if not, whether empathetic interfaces can help. According to an in-depth RAND Corporation report released in mid-2013, many wellness programs are ineffective. [63] For example:

- People participating in wellness initiatives only lost an average of one pound per year over a three-year period.
- Employers express confidence that workplace wellness programs lower health costs; however, RAND found that organizations rarely measure them and wellness plans only save employers an average of $157 per participant.

Another major issue is the fact that many people who are eligible for wellness programs either do not participate or drop out. Some of the reasons RAND found employees did not participate included "long wait times and rigid work schedules." [63]

Despite the questions surrounding workplace wellness programs, they are not going away. Can technology help employers measure them more effectively, boost participation, and promote engagement? Some digital health companies are betting that empathetic interfaces, predictive analytics, and other tools can improve the effectiveness of wellness initiatives.

Healthrageous is one firm that has integrated a range of these technologies into its wellness solutions. The company, which was sold to insurance firm Humana in October 2013, developed a digital health management platform used by employers and health plans.[3] [64] At the center of Healthrageous's tool is a mobile app-delivered intelligent digital health coach. Rather than peppering users with a series of generic health messages, the coach provides education and encouragement in friendly, understandable, human language. Healthrageous's technology also utilizes data collected via sensing devices (re: blood pressure, physical activity, etc.) to personalize users' experiences and deliver daily encouragement.

In addition to providing a personable digital health coach, Healthrageous's app ups the human factor by helping users connect with others to either receive encouragement or provide support. The company's technology also features predictive analytics tools that further personalize the health messages participants receive and may prevent people from leaving the wellness program.

Recap: How Empathetic Interfaces May Help Save Money in Health

As described above, empathetic interfaces are helping hospitals reduce readmission rates and may improve the effectiveness of wellness programs. These tools can also help hospitals and employers reduce health spending by:

- **Facilitating Care Management Outside the Hospital:** Telemedicine tools (with empathetic interfaces), supported by predictive analytics, may help prevent re-hospitalization and reduce costs. Health providers can use these technologies to identify which patients are at highest risk of becoming ill and proactively communicate with them using telemedicine technologies.
- **Improving Employees' Engagement With Wellness Programs:** Developing engaging, responsive, and personalized digital wellness programs powered by empathetic interfaces may increase the odds employees actually participate in these initiatives. In addition, using health data collected via sensors can help employees monitor their progress and make health messages more relevant and persuasive. Finally, analytics may enable employers to make data-influenced decisions about which elements of wellness initiatives are actually reducing medical expenses and improving health.

Do ePatients Believe Empathetic Interfaces Could Improve Their Health?

The ultimate empathetic interface would be a human-like computer avatar (or virtual person) that provides ongoing advice, support, and information to patients, caregivers, and others. (Below we provide an example of a company that is currently developing and deploying this type of digital health technology.) Given this, we were especially interested in understanding whether ePatients believe that this type of empathetic health support and educational system would be beneficial or encourage them to engage in healthier behaviors.

To find out, Enspektos asked ePatients participating in the 2013 edition of its digihealth pulse study whether they believed technologies or devices featuring animated or computer-generated people (better known as avatars), rather than text or video, could improve their health or willingness to exercise, lose weight, or engage in other positive health behaviors.[4]

We learned that many ePatients would welcome health tools featuring this type of empathetic interface. Half of ePatients told us they believe devices or technologies featuring human-like interfaces would benefit their health or motivate them to eat better, exercise, or do something else that would improve their wellbeing (Figure III).

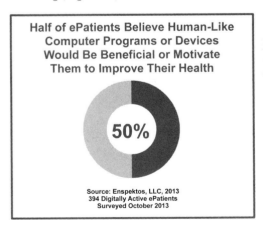

Half of ePatients Believe Human-Like Computer Programs or Devices Would Be Beneficial or Motivate Them to Improve Their Health

50%

Source: Enspektos, LLC, 2013
394 Digitally Active ePatients
Surveyed October 2013

Figure III: Percentage of ePatients Who Feel Empathetic Interfaces Featuring Animated or Computer-Generated People Would Help Them Engage in Positive Health Behaviors or Have Other Benefits

This suggests that ePatients are willing to accept, and would be potentially motivated by, technologies that are more personable, empathetic, responsive, and human.

Stories: Empathetic Interfaces

HealthTxts: A Mobile Health Intervention With a Human Touch

It is notoriously difficult for people to change set behaviors, and this fact leads to all kinds of health problems—from unhealthy eating habits to low- or non-adherence to prescribed medications. The insight behind HealthTxts, founded by Columbia University behavioral psychologist Dr. Fred Muench in 2009, was that text messages can drive immediate behavior change because of the real-time nature of the message, the tendency for people to check text messages immediately (as opposed to e-mails) and the ability to personalize messages based on individual preferences.

HealthTxts offers a combination of personalized messages as well as human-developed advice from medical professionals. Perhaps the true reason HealthTxts has been successful at changing behavior, is due to its real-time empathetic interface specifically built to align with how people actually live their daily lives. In a recent study of the program, 80% of people receiving the messages reported that they served as good reminders of why they wanted to change their behavior. And, 81% chose to continue receiving HealthTxts messages after the pilot was over.

Learn More: http://www.healthtxts.com/why-it-works

Enroll UX 2014: Using Human-Centered Interface Design to Help People Purchase Health Insurance Coverage

About a year before the Affordable Care Act was rolled out in the United States, a public-private partnership between eight national and state health care foundations was created to tackle what was already predicted to be a huge user interface challenge. The global design and innovation consultancy IDEO was selected by the sponsoring foundations to lead the initiative to adopt a "human-centered, design-based approach" to research and recommend best design practices for an "online health insurance portal that will make it easier for people to understand the coverage they may be eligible for and will support their enrollment decision-making." [65]

A seemingly robust set of templates and guides was delivered in June of 2013, but was not implemented due to a combination of overblown expectations and the inability to execute the recommendations. When user experience architect Rob Condit reviewed its failure, he noted that the entire project "was—and remains—a vastly powerful toolkit that provides a pan-industry model of Web site excellence and offers us an abundance of tools to extend and develop further. The rest is up to us." [66]

Learn More: http://www.ux2014.org

Vitality GlowCap: An Empathetic Prescription Bottle Cap Reminds People to Take Their Medications

Another innovative firm offering a solution to the common problem of medical adherence is Vitality. Their product, branded as GlowCap, promises to "remember so you don't have to." The product is a replacement cap that fits on top of a standard prescription bottle and that visually glows when it is time to take medicine. The cap is also integrated with optional wireless communication, so the bottle can automatically reorder pills when patients are running low.

As Dr. Joseph Cafazzo, lead of the Centre for Global eHealth Innovation, noted in 2013, "There is a vital need for empathy in design if the use of medical devices is to succeed in homes and other nontraditional environments." The Vitality GlowCap succeeds in this mission with innovation, empathy, and functionality. [67]

The global mainstream media has widely covered the GlowCap, and it has become one of the most celebrated and simple health-care innovations of the last several years.

Learn More: http://www.vitality.net

---

[3] Humana may incorporate Healthrageous's technologies into its own wellness program-related offerings.
[4] See Appendix I for more information about digihealth pulse.

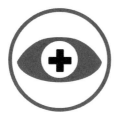

Trend 2:
Unhealthy Surveillance

The rapid rise of surveillance technologies that combine clinical and behavioral data to monitor the health of individuals and groups of people presents significant privacy and security concerns. The volume of tools and informaton being developed and collected vastly outstrips the ability of regulators and policymakers to understand and react to it in time to prevent the potential for misuse.

Steve Howe is CEO of Acxiom Corporation, a marketing technology firm that has collected massive amounts of data about most American adults. Acxiom analyzes the personal information it collects for a range of purposes, including helping Facebook deliver more personalized and relevant ads to people. [68]

Given Howe's knowledge of his company's activities, you wouldn't expect him to be surprised about the data Acxiom possesses about him, but he was. After entering his personal details into a public Web site maintained by Acxiom and released in early September 2013 called AboutTheData.com, Howe learned that the firm knows the size of his house, that he's interested in tennis, and is a regular domestic traveler. [69]

Howe told the *New York Times* he decided to have Acxiom develop the site partly to alleviate fears about the vast amounts of personal data being collected about Americans. He also hopes to prepare his firm for the day when government may seek to more aggressively regulate the activities of data brokers like Acxiom. [69]

Acxiom is not only collecting information about Americans' retail purchases and mortgages. Health is also an area of focus. For example, users of AbouttheData.com can find out what Acxiom knows about their recent health activities such as whether they purchased cholesterol products. [69]

Has the health industry been participating in the intense data privacy debate currently consuming executives from government, advertising agencies, technology companies, and other organizations? Yes, to some degree; however, health organizations have long focused on privacy issues, partly because securing health data has always been a major concern. One reason is because private health information is already heavily protected under a U.S. law called HIPAA.[5] This legislation mandates that health insurance companies, providers, and health-care clearinghouses (companies that facilitate health billing and other administrative tasks) responsible for handling patients' personally identifiable information must take steps to store it securely and protect if from unauthorized access.

HIPPA has a giant loophole, though. Organizations and individuals who are not "covered entities" (health insurance companies, health-care providers, and health-care clearinghouses), but still handling sensitive health information are exempt from the law's requirements. [70]

Recently, federal regulators have taken steps to narrow this loophole. For example, partly in response to major privacy violations, the U.S. Department of Health and Human Services released a new rule in January 2013 designed to "improve privacy protections and security safeguards for consumer health data." [71] Among other things, the rule extends HIPPA's privacy requirements to "business associates of these [covered] entities that receive protected health information, such as contractors and subcontractors." [71]

This new rule suggests that government officials are starting to pay more attention to the fact that a growing numbers of companies, individuals, and others are collecting, storing, and selling personal health information; however, much more needs to be done to protect consumers' private health information. In an interview conducted for this book, Jody Ranck, digital health futurist and author of *Connected Health: How Mobile Phones, Cloud, and Big Data Will Reinvent Healthcare*, told us he is concerned about "secondary data players" who are "unaccustomed to dealing with health data." He warns that "established health-care players could get burnt" if they are sloppy about how they work with companies that are not covered by HIPPA, but collecting and providing personal health information.

Who are secondary data players? These organizations include social networks, mobile health application developers, and health device makers. Hackers also pose a threat to health data privacy—and may even threaten lives. When we talk about the privacy and security problems associated with "unhealthy surveillance" our focus is on these groups. Following is a brief overview of some health privacy threats associated with data collected (or breeched) by secondary data players.

Clicking Facebook's Like Button Could Reveal More Than You Think

Clicking (or tapping) Facebook's Like button is easy and fun. But would people be less willing to Like something if they knew this information could be used to learn intimate details about them? In 2013, researchers revealed how they can analyze data about people's Likes on Facebook to:

- **Determine Who is Most Likely to Be Overweight:** Researchers at the Harvard School of Public Health have discovered that if you Like television programs on Facebook you may be more likely to be overweight than those who do not. For example, people living in the Northeast Bronx were more apt to Like television shows. Publicly available data suggests Bronx dwellers are also more likely to be overweight. The opposite was true for those living in low overweight, high physical activity areas of the country such as Coeur d'Alene, Idaho. People from these regions were more likely to Like exercise-related activities versus TV programs. [72, 73]

- **Predict Personal Characteristics and Unhealthy Behaviors:** In another study published in 2013, researchers were able to correctly determine users' sexual orientation, race, and a range of health behaviors, including tobacco and drug use by analyzing Facebook Like data.[6] [74]

While using Facebook Like data to track and predict health status and behavior may have public health benefits, there is also the potential for abuse. Most importantly, this information could be collected and used without Facebook users' consent to reveal intimate details about them, guide unwanted marketing activities, and more.

Health Data Provided by Mobile App Users is Being Shared Without Their Knowledge or Consent

Mobile health and fitness applications are very popular, but are users and app developers paying enough attention to security and privacy? Perhaps not, according to a 2013 study released by the Privacy Rights Clearinghouse. [75] The group found that developers of mobile health apps routinely share user data with outside groups, such as advertisers, without users' knowledge or consent. Free applications were the least privacy protecting; however, premium app developers still engage in questionable practices. Among paid mobile health apps studied by the Clearinghouse:

- 30% shared users' data with organizations not listed in apps' privacy policies
- Only 10% secured data sent from the application to developers
- Less than half (44%) of paid apps encrypted personally identifiable user data transmitted to developers or third parties

Although mobile health app developers are not paying enough attention to user privacy or doing enough to secure health information they are sharing, the Clearinghouse did not recommend people stop using these products; instead, they suggested mobile users think carefully before doing so. [75]

Hackers Are Accessing Private Health Information and Could Breech Medical Devices, or Shut Them Down

The reason the Privacy Rights Clearinghouse focused so much on data encryption is because of the risk that hackers and other non-authorized individuals could access highly sensitive health data from mobile applications; however, mobile health apps are not the only health technology vulnerable to hackers.

For example, in 2012 the U.S. Office for Civil Rights reported that more than 21 million people's personal health data had been compromised since 2009. The majority of data breaches were due to theft while 6% were blamed on hackers. [76, 77]

In addition, security experts have demonstrated how medical devices such as pacemakers can be hacked and shut down remotely. [78] Hospitals are also battling a range of viruses and malware that have infected their computers. [79]

Web Users' Health Searches Are Being Shared With Others

In a July 2013 research letter published in *JAMA Internal Medicine*, Dr. Marco Huesch revealed that seven of the 20 popular health Web sites he examined shared information about users' sensitive search queries with third parties. [80] While U.S. government Web sites refrained from sharing user data, other properties, including the *New York Times*, Drugs.com, and the United Kingdom's National Health Service site did so. [80] In response to this report, Lisa Madigan, the attorney general of Illinois, sent letters to eight health Web sites asking for more information about their data use polices and practices. [81]

Sensitive Health Data Collected via Wearable Devices Could Be Accidently Shared

In July 2011, *The Next Web* reported that users of Fitbit's personal tracking device were inadvertently posting sensitive information about their sex lives to Google. [82] This was because many Fitbit users had not changed a default privacy setting on the device's Web site that shared their health data with everyone by default. Fitbit was quick to block this information from public display, but the incident revealed what can happen when wearable device makers don't think carefully enough about user privacy and security. [83]

The examples listed above are just a few of the privacy issues that are gaining attention due to the vast amounts of health data being collected and shared on mobile devices, social media, and elsewhere. Yet the question still remains: Do people actually care about health data privacy? In the area of non-health data, many believe the answer is no. This is because revelations that companies such as Google and Facebook are collecting personal data (and sharing it with governments around the world) has not lead to a mass exodus from tools developed by these companies; however, a 2013 poll conducted by Microsoft suggests that many people may not be leaving these services due to a sense they have "little or no control over the personal information companies gather about them." [84]

While the debate about whether consumers care about digital privacy issues will continue, there is little doubt that health is different. People may be more concerned about how their health data is collected and used—especially regarding conditions they may not wish to be revealed such as their mental health or STD status. This is one of the reasons why we took a closer look at whether ePatients are worried about unhealthy surveillance.

Are ePatients Concerned About Unhealthy Surveillance?

As discussed above, many different organizations are collecting and sharing health data. Given this, Enspektos asked ePatients participating in the 2013 edition of its digihealth pulse study to rate their level of concern that their personal health information might be collected and shared without their consent.[7] Personal health data could include details about foods they purchased, health content they shared on social networks, medical keywords typed into search engines, and more. ePatients used a five-point scale where 1 = Low Concern 3 = Moderate Concern and 5 = Very High Concern.

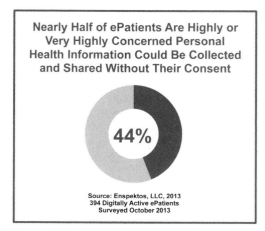

Nearly Half of ePatients Are Highly or Very Highly Concerned Personal Health Information Could Be Collected and Shared Without Their Consent

44%

Source: Enspektos, LLC, 2013
394 Digitally Active ePatients
Surveyed October 2013

Figure IV: Percentage of ePatients Concerned that Personal Health Information from Digital Channels Could be Collected or Shared Without Their Consent

Enspektos found that many (44%) of ePatients are highly or very highly concerned about health data privacy (Figure IV).[8] This data indicates that regulators, device manufacturers, companies producing social networks, and others should be thinking carefully about how to ensure that users are informed about what personal health data is being collected, how it is being used, and the steps being taken to prevent unauthorized use of this information.

Stories: Unhealthy Surveillance

Harvard University's Data Privacy Lab Researches the Scope of Unhealthy Surveillance

One of the reassuring "truths" that we are often told about our health data is that it is sometimes recorded anonymously or in aggregate without specific references to our personal details. Yet as former Google CEO Eric Schmidt once creepily noted, "With your permission . . . we know where you are. We know where you've been. We can more or less know what you're thinking about." [85]

As several research projects from the Data Privacy Lab run by Harvard Professor of Government and Technology in Residence Dr. Latanya Sweeney have uncovered, there are myriad ways that data can be reverse-engineered to uncover personal details you assumed would be private or unassociated with your health data. As a result, organizations and people with sometimes far more evil motives than Google may be able to use this information to do harm.

Learn More: http://dataprivacylab.org/people/sweeney/

Conducting Health Surveillance from Inside the Body: Proteus Digital Health's Ingestible, Sensing Pills

Some of the benefits of "digital medicines" include their ability to capture and share data about how medications are working in your body, offer recommendations to improve their efficacy, and send reminders to keep patients taking drugs as prescribed. Proteus Digital Health has developed a sensing device that can be incorporated into prescription medications that, once swallowed, provides a wealth of health data from inside the body.

On the surface, Proteus' product seems like a perfect solution to improve health care—but there is a potential downside. These "smart pills" can be used to share data with doctors and insurance companies, potentially without patients' knowledge. This is a perfect example of the simultaneous potential benefits and risks associated with capturing patient data from inside the body.

Learn More: http://www.proteus.com/future-products/digital-medicines/

CVS ExtraCare Rewards Program: Offering Perks in Exchange for Private Wellness and Health Data

This leading U.S. drugstore chain has pioneered a loyalty program that millions of consumers are actively using each day to earn points in exchange for cash rewards or discounts on products. The program provides significant rewards in exchange for customers' willingness to give up their private data. What seems like a fair trade to most consumers, though, may not seem so if this private information is shared with third parties for the purpose of targeting marketing or other reasons.

Learn More: http://articles.latimes.com/2013/aug/15/business/la-fi-lazarus-20130816

---

[5] HIPPA stands for the Health Insurance Portability and Accountability Act of 1996.

[6] If you'd like to see what your Facebook Likes say about you, visit www.youarewhatyoulike.com. No information about your health behaviors and activities will be displayed, but you can view interesting information about your personality and habits.

[7] See Appendix I for more information about digihealth pulse.

[8] Percentage of ePatients selecting 4 (highly concerned) and 5 (very highly concerned) shown in Figure IV.

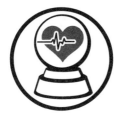

Trend 3:
Predictive Psychohistory

In Isaac Asimov's "Foundation" series mathematics, politics and history combine to enable "psychohistorians" to predict future events. In the real world, Big Data, powerful computer algorithms, and more are being used to make large- and small-scale predictions about individual and population health. We are entering the age of health psychohistory.

The late scientist, author and futurist Isaac Asimov, is credited with shaping the rise of a number of scientific fields such as robotics. Many of the technologies he discussed in his science fiction novels evolved significantly during his lifetime; however, there was one concept he developed called psychohistory that he never imagined might one day become a reality—although in an altered form.

In the non-fiction realm, *psychohistory* is a historical field focused on the study of past events from a psychological perspective. Psychohistory was especially popular during the 1930s and psychohistorians regularly published articles designed to uncover the hidden motivations behind the actions of key historical figures such as Edgar Alan Poe and Julius Caesar. [86]

Asimov was aware of the term psychohistory and decided to incorporate the word into his *Foundation* series of science fiction stories, although in a different manner. In a 1987 interview broadcast on National Public Radio's *Fresh Air*, Asimov revealed his motivation for developing his version of psychohistory, saying: "I assumed that the time would come when there would be a science in which things could be predicted on a probabilistic or statistical basis." [87]

Asimov's psychohistory has the following characteristics:

1. Statistics can be used to determine (based on data about past historical events) the probable future actions of large groups of people
2. Psychohistory cannot predict the actions of individuals, only large populations
3. The general population cannot be made aware of events predicted using psychohistorical mathematical techniques

When asked perhaps the most important question about psychohistory by *Fresh Air's* host Terry Gross—"whether it would be good if there really was such as science," Asimov replied, "I can't help but think it would be." [87]

Like so much of his other remarkably prescient thinking, in the decades after his death in 1992 technology has indeed advanced to the point where we now have the ability to collect and analyze large amounts of historical health data and make predictions about the future wellbeing of large groups—and individuals. The age of predictive health psychohistory has arrived.

Data, Mathematics and Learning Machines:
The Building Blocks of Health Psychohistory

These days we often hear about the promise of Big Data analytics to enable us to quickly and accurately analyze large and diverse data sets of all kinds. While other areas such as finance and digital generate large amounts of information, health is especially data rich. With each heartbeat, the human body generates vast amounts of information on everything from blood pressure to brain function. Doctors regularly capture high-resolution videos and images of organs and other body parts. Patients leave robust data trails when filling prescriptions via mobile, searching for medical information online, and more. Our individual and collective health histories are made up of the types of data described above. Today, we are learning to use powerful machines along with mathematics to predict who will get sick, experience a depressive episode, fail to take medications as prescribed, and more. In fact, as we collect better data and recognize deeper connections, our health-related predictions may become more accurate.

Describing the art and science of using data to predict health behavior and outcomes—what we refer to as predictive psychohistory—generally consists of:

- **Collecting Diverse Information:** Without data it would be impossible to make predictions. Gathering data from as many sources as possible is also important. In fact, Dr. Alan Greene, chief medical officer of Scanadu, a firm developing a series of health sensors for the consumer market, has noted that many types of what we tend to think as non-health information can have a bearing on our wellbeing. [88] For example, researchers working at the Harvard School of Public Health analyzed Kenyans' travel activities (based on data collected via mobile devices) and uncovered a surprising link to the spread of malaria. They found that people who traveled outside the town of Kericho were also highly likely to visit Lake Victoria, a well-known malaria hot spot. [89]

- **Training the Machines:** Data is only the fuel for the predictive machine. Computer programs designed to perform a range of mathematical calculations are its engine. These programs not only analyze data, but learn from it. The process used to educate computer programs is called machine learning. In order for machines to learn effectively, they must be presented with a diverse range of data, or variables, that can be used to calculate the likelihood of future events.

- **Generating Predictive Models:** Eric Siegel author of *Predictive Analytics: The Power to Predict Who Will Click, Buy, Lie, or Die*, provides a particularly clear explanation of how predictive models are designed. According to Siegel, predictive models use the "characteristics (variables) of the individual as input, and provides a predictive score as output. The higher the score, the more likely it is that the individual will exhibit the predicted behavior." [21]

Two Ways Predictive Psychohistory May Help Reduce Health Spending

Beyond improving outcomes or care, predictive tools can have a particularly powerful effect when it comes to addressing the challenge of reducing health spending. Two of the cost-saving benefits of health psychohistory are briefly outlined below.

1. **Prevent Major Health Events:** If we can predict when people are likely to have a heart attack, enter a major depressive episode, or experience another health event, we can intervene earlier, save lives, and potentially reduce spending. This is what Ginger.io and those working with this digital health startup hope to achieve. Ginger.io has developed a mobile application that serves as a "check engine light" for hospitals and other organizations managing the health of large groups of people. The company collects a range of data emitted by people's mobile phones, including how many calls they make, whether they are traveling or not, and survey information provided by those who have downloaded their mobile app. This information is then used to help doctors, insurance companies, and others anticipate when people are not doing well and contact them proactively. Connecting with people before they enter the hospital may reduce medical spending and improve the way health providers manage care. [90]

2. **Reducing Medical Errors:** Patients rely on doctors to diagnose their conditions accurately, but what if physicians make the wrong diagnosis? Even worse, what are the consequences for patients if they receive a prescription for the incorrect medication? Unfortunately, medical errors are all too common. In 1999, the Institute of Medicine (IOM) reported that nearly 100,000 people die of medical errors each year. [91] In addition to lives lost, mistakes are expensive. In its 1999 report, the IOM estimated that errors cost hospitals, patients, and others nearly $29 billion per year. [91] Unfortunately, more than a decade after IOM's report, medical errors are still a major problem. Thankfully, Big Data can help.

IBM's super computer, Watson, best known for defeating humans in Jeopardy, is being used in health care. Watson utilizes a range of data analytics technologies to measure and predict which treatment options are best for individual patients. According to Dr. Martin Kohn, chief medical scientist at IBM Research, Watson is not designed to replace doctors, but help them diagnose disease accurately, select treatments based on scientific evidence, and reduce medical errors, especially those related to prescription drugs. [47] Watson is not only for physicians, but can be used by patients to help them make better decisions about their care, especially in complex and serious conditions such as cancer. [47]

The age of predictive psychohistory in health is still in its infancy; yet, it has the potential to profoundly influence how care is delivered, patients are treated, and much more. Following are a few more stories that illustrate how predictive psychohistory is taking shape today.

Stories: Predictive Psychohistory

RxAnte Reveals Who is Most Likely to Stop Taking Medications

RxAnte is one of several innovative companies using predictive analytics to uncover which patients are most likely to stop taking medications. By collecting vast amounts of data and analyzing multiple variables, the company helps health plans, providers, and companies deliver interventions just-in-time to keep people from discontinuing needed medications.

Learn More: http://www.rxante.com

The Dutch Health Hub Predicts Breast Cancer Using Raw Imaging Data

The city of Almere in the Netherlands has created an ambitious program known as Almere DataCapital, which aims to harness the potential of data analytics by "building an eco-system of companies, education, and research facilities that will provide knowledge and services about and for Big Data." [92]

The program's first project is the Dutch Health Hub, a public and private partnership that makes raw health data available for clinical and research purposes. One of the first efforts of this hub, for example, uses a combination of algorithms and computing power to detect breast cancer sooner using a breast scan's raw data to analyze tissue density and anomalies *before* it is converted to an image. Other research efforts are currently in progress.

Learn More: http://www.almeredatacapital.nl/index.php?option=com_content&view=article&id=68&Itemid=255

IBM STEM: Using Big Data to Predict the Next Global Pandemic

If the global plague often predicted by Hollywood disaster films ever happens, the good news is we may have a fighting chance of actually predicting it—or at least understanding how it may spread. For years, IBM has been working on a tool known as the Spatio-Temporal Epidemiological Modeler (which thankfully goes by the acronym STEM). It is being made freely available by the Eclipse Foundation to help scientists and others create and use models of infectious diseases and how they may evolve over time. The aim of the project is to help grow worldwide understanding of diseases such as Avian Flu and Salmonella and potentially prevent or contain their spread.

Learn More: http://ibmresearchnews.blogspot.com/2009/09/guest-blog-can-we-forecast-next.html
http://www.almaden.ibm.com/cs/projects/stem

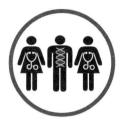

Part 2:
The Personalized Health Movement:
Using Technology, Data, Genetics, and More to Escape Generic Medicine

"This is a new era of medicine, in which each person can be near fully defined at the individual level, instead of how we [currently] practice medicine, [which is] at a population level . . ."

– Dr. Eric Topol, *The Creative Destruction of Medicine: How the Digital Revolution Will Create Better Health Care* [32]

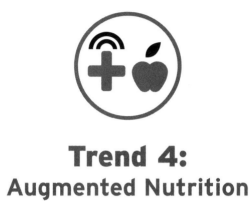

Trend 4:
Augmented Nutrition

In a quest to better understand what is going into their bodies, consumers are turning to a range of tools and technologies that provide augmented nutritional information on food products to help them make healthful choices about what they buy and eat. Access to real-time augmented nutrition information during retail purchase and restaurant dining situations is also allowing for deeper product comparisons and impacting purchase behavior.

Is First Lady Michelle Obama a quiet food revolutionary? Mark Hertsgaard, a fellow at the New America Foundation and co-founder of the environmental group Climate Parents, thinks so. Writing in *The Nation* in 2009 shortly after Obama began planting an organic garden on the South Lawn of the White House, Hertsgaard called the act of advocating home-grown food "subversive" because it raises awareness that "the food most Americans eat nowadays is not fresh, tasty, or healthy." [93]

Eric Schlosser, who wrote the surprise best seller *Fast Food Nation*, also views Obama's garden as a watershed moment in the American food landscape. In *Fast Food Nation*, Schlosser describes how mass food is produced, while highlighting some of the ways it harms the environment and our bodies. [94] Writing in the *Daily Beast* in 2012, Schlosser talked about how his book (combined with the work of other authors, filmmakers, and journalists) helped make an organic garden at the White House possible rather than "inconceivable." [95]

Schlosser placed Obama's efforts in the context of a global food movement that has emerged and strengthened over the past fifteen years or so. This movement is defined by an emphasis on understanding how food is produced and helping to support the production and consumption of environmentally and body-friendly foods (e.g., locally grown produce, organic foods, etc.).

At its heart, the steadily expanding food movement is about knowledge and control. In the past, most consumers ceded control to government, agriculture, and food companies and spent little time considering the health and environmental consequences of their dietary decisions. Today, a growing number of people are gathering more information about what they eat and demanding greater accountability from themselves and those responsible for keeping the global food engine running.

The Augmented Nutrition trend can be viewed as a natural outgrowth of the food movement's emphasis on knowledge and control. People are turning to digital technologies to help them make more informed (and personalized) dietary decisions based on access to more transparent information about food's health and environmental impacts. Given the link between Augmented Nutrition and beliefs and practices that started within the food movement, it makes sense to briefly summarize its history and scope.

Convenience, Politics, and Control: A Brief History of the Food Movement in America

As noted earlier in this book, the United States (along with other nations) is experiencing an epidemic of conditions such as Type II diabetes and heart disease. Many of these diseases can be prevented or treated with diet. For example, in 1997 researchers published a study in the *New England Journal of Medicine* suggesting that a low-sodium diet rich in fruits, vegetables, and low-fat dairy products can reduce high blood pressure. [96]

Because eating a healthful diet is so important, many are asking why it is so difficult for people to break bad dietary habits. In her book, *How America Eats: A Social History of U.S. Food and Culture,* Jennifer Jensen Wallach suggests culture may be to blame. She writes: "From the beginning of European colonization, settlers wished to eat more abundantly and to eat more animal protein than generations before them...This sense of culinary entitlement has been a defining feature of American food culture as each generation has measured its well-being by the large quantities, particularly of meat, that it could consume." [97]

Wallach also asserts that "habit and history" have a greater influence on food choices than "recommendations from doctors and nutritionists." [97] In addition, she suggests government, corporations, and the agriculture industry have responded to Americans' cultural emphasis on abundance by developing policies, practices, and technologies designed to make food more available and convenient to cook and consume. [97]

Partly, because the food industry has succeeded in making what we eat cheap, plentiful, and convenient, many people living in Western cultures (and to a growing degree, Eastern cultures as well) have been largely apathetic about the consequences (both positive and negative) of the industrial techniques used to produce and deliver what we eat. Despite this, journalists, novelists, and others have succeeded in raising awareness and concern about how food is manufactured from time to time over the last century.

Perhaps the most widely known example comes from 1906, when "muckraking" journalist Upton Sinclair's novel *The Jungle* was first published. Based on Sinclair's experiences working undercover in a meat-packing plant, *The Jungle* describes how food delivered to homes across the nation was pumped full of chemicals, produced in unsanitary conditions, and even sometimes contaminated with human body parts. [98] Sinclair's book shocked the nation and helped to secure the passage of the Pure Food and Drug Act of 1906, which led to the formation of the modern day U.S. Food and Drug Administration. [97]

Over the next century, the public's confidence in food manufacturing steadily increased. In that time, economic and social factors (including efforts to lower the cost of labor and an increase in immigration) also resulted in the consolidation of the global food industry and boosted its ability to deliver food cheaply. [94] Consumption of fast food accelerated as public scrutiny of the food industry dramatically decreased.

A radical shift, according to best selling food author Michael Pollan, finally came in the late 1980s when "a series of food safety scandals opened people's eyes to the way their food was being produced, each one drawing the curtain back a little further on a food system that had changed beyond recognition." [99]

In the next few decades, a greater focus on food production, safety, and health steadily crept into media reports, best selling books, documentary films, and pop culture. This content helped to form the inspiration and intellectual underpinnings for the growing global food movement.

In summary, the core of the food movement can be boiled down to a quest for two things: knowledge and control.

1. Having the knowledge to understand where the food you consume comes from, how it was produced, what it is doing to your body, and how best to prepare it
2. The ability to control how you eat and do so in ways that align with your personal wellness, ethical and political beliefs and goals

ePatients and the Food Movement

So how does the global food movement connect with ePatients? With an eye toward understanding how ePatients perceive certain issues critical to those in the food movement, Enspektos looked at whether they believe it is important to purchase and cook organic food in the 2012 edition of its digihealth pulse study (see Appendix I for more about this research). Some of the survey data Enspektos collected from ePatients on this topic is shown in Figures V and VI.

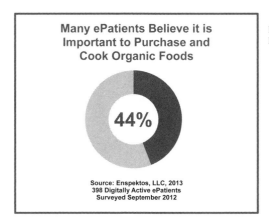

Many ePatients Believe it is Important to Purchase and Cook Organic Foods

44%

Source: Enspektos, LLC, 2013
398 Digitally Active ePatients
Surveyed September 2012

Figure V: Percentage of ePatients Who Believe Organic Foods Are Important

Enspektos found that nearly half (44%) of ePatients believe it is important to purchase and cook organic foods (Figure V). Even more interesting (and perhaps illustrating how much the food movement has become embedded in the American cultural landscape), 50% of ePatients making $30,000 or less also feel organic foods are important (Figure VI).

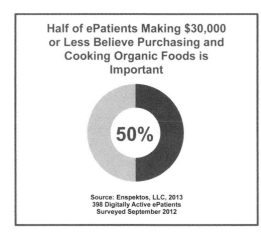

Half of ePatients Making $30,000 or Less Believe Purchasing and Cooking Organic Foods is Important

50%

Source: Enspektos, LLC, 2013
398 Digitally Active ePatients
Surveyed September 2012

Figure VI: Percentage of Low-Income ePatients Who Believe Organic Foods Are Important

How Augmented Nutrition Technologies Help People Gain Knowledge and Control

Digital Augmented Nutrition technologies can help people radically transform their eating habits and spread the food movement's beliefs and practices to broader segments of the public by:

- **Broadening Knowledge About Food:** Gathering information about the food we eat can be a difficult process. Food labels provide limited information and much of the food we eat is consumed or purchased in places where it is hard to conduct research. Digital tools, such as mobile applications, can help people gather food data on the go and when they are making decisions about what to buy and eat.
- **Boosting Control Over Food Choices:** As discussed above, powerful cultural and social forces contribute to overeating and poor diet. Digital technologies, especially if they place people in contact with others who share their values and beliefs about food, may aid in the development and maintenance of healthful eating habits.
- **Informing Real-Time Food Decisions:** Given the rising role of technology in consumer behavior, smartphones are bringing information and knowledge into the critical last-mile moment when consumers are standing in front of store shelves and deciding what to buy. As more information becomes instantly available at their fingertips, it is starting to impact their purchase decisions in powerful ways.

Let's look at a few more stories of how the Augmented Nutrition trend is affecting the food people buy and what they eat.

Stories: Augmented Nutrition

The Fooducate Plus App Delivers Augmented Nutritional Information to "Always On" Consumers

Of the dozens of smartphone apps available that help people track their diets and food options, one of the most popular (as of this writing) is an app called Fooducate Plus. This application allows consumers to set up simple profiles and scan images of foods they have purchased or are considering buying.

In addition to linking these foods to online health tracking devices and accounts, the app provides real-time assessments of their nutritional value and even suggests alternatives that may be more healthful. This real-time tracking and information at people's fingertips is a concept being explored and executed against by countless apps that are targeting people described by Experian's United Kingdom research arm as "always on consumers." [100] For this audience, Augmented Nutrition is rapidly evolving from a luxury item to an essential tool.

Learn More: http://www.fooducate.com

Toronto Public Health Helps People Make More Healthful Choices Using Improved Food Labeling

When it comes to restaurant meals, one of the hottest topics in the global debate is the food's healthfulness or lack thereof. Some cities around the world have adopted legislation requiring large restaurant chains to display calorie counts on menus. Toronto Public Health, however, has taken the debate one step further. With programs such as its Savvy Diner campaign, they go beyond the basic calorie counts and encourage restaurants to provide better menu labeling regarding all kinds of nutritional information, including fat content and sodium. With an increasing array of research, which demonstrates that better menu labeling promotes food transparency and more healthful eating, this issue and initiatives like the one launched by Toronto Public Health, will continue to resonate and accelerate through 2015 and beyond.

Learn More:
http://www.toronto.ca/health/nutrition/menu_labelling.htm
http://www.savvydiner.ca/

Pictrition Builds a Global Virtual Community Dedicated to Helping People Understand What They Eat

In October of 2013, Austin-based startup Loop Health was invited to debut their newest product at the prestigious DEMO conference—the same event where Netflix and E-trade launched. The product they demonstrated was based on the innovative idea that tracking the food you eat shouldn't involve searching through complex databases or being forced to enter detailed nutritional information; instead, Pictrition allows users to snap a photo of their meal, and get instant nutritional feedback from Pictrition's community of "pictritionists." Perhaps more importantly, the tool gamifies the process of keeping a food journal, which most nutritionists and weight loss consultants agree is a critical first step towards starting and maintaining a more healthful lifestyle.[9]

Learn More: http://loophealth.co/#pictrition

---

[9] See trend 12, MicroHealth Rewards, for more information about gamification.

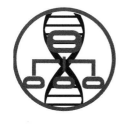

Trend 5:
Medical Genealogy

Genomics and advances in digital genealogy will combine, allowing patients to use their ancestral and genetic history to predict the risk of disease and, more importantly, how they may respond to medications. This data may one day become a valuable asset to pass on to future generations.

Could genetics explain why African Americans are more likely to develop late-onset Alzheimer's disease, or LOAD, than people of European ancestry? Answering this question is important because LOAD is a common cause of dementia in seniors, especially among those 80-plus years of age. [101]

In 2013, researchers published an analysis of genetic data collected from nearly 6,000 African Americans, aged 60 years and older (with and without LOAD) in the medical journal *JAMA*. [101] Scientists identified key sets of genetic variations (or mutations) in blacks that appear to increase the risk for LOAD.[10] When comparing data collected and analyzed for this study (and previously among patients of European descent), Alzheimer's patients of African American and European ancestry both had variations at the ABCA7 gene; however, despite sharing the same ABCA7 variation with whites, this genetic mutation appeared to put African Americans at *significantly higher* risk for LOAD. [101]

This research is important because there have been fewer genetic studies conducted among people from ethnic and racial minority groups. Like in the case of the LOAD study discussed above, researchers are learning that while people from various ancestral backgrounds may share certain genetic characteristics, their risk of developing certain diseases may be different. Scientists have also discovered that genetic differences between people may influence how they respond to medications.

The *JAMA* study discussed above is a prime example of Medical Genealogy: the art and science of using information about people's ethnic/family background *in combination* with their genetic profile to predict disease and influence how drugs are prescribed. In this chapter, we focus on the implications of Medical Genealogy for patients, caregivers, and families given the recent rapid rise in personal genetic testing, which is discussed below.

From Spit in a Cup to Disease Risk Prediction: Understanding Personal Genetic Testing

Imagine you are one of the most successful technology entrepreneurs on the planet. Your inventions have transformed humanity; you possess billions in personal wealth, and are fit enough to participate in world-class athletic events. Life seems perfect . . . until you take a genetic test and learn you have a very high chance of developing a devastating disease with no cure.

This was the situation Sergey Brin, co-founder of Google, found himself in after he had his genetic material analyzed as an early customer (and investor) of 23andMe, a personal genetic testing company. His wife, Anne Wojcicki (who co-founded 23andMe), encouraged him to check and see whether he had a mutation in his LRRK2 gene called G2019S. Some studies suggest that people who have the G2019S mutation are at a significantly higher risk of Parkinson's. Brin learned that he has this mutation. His mother, who also has it, developed Parkinson's earlier in her life. [102]

Brin faced a situation many more people will confront in the near future as personal genetic testing becomes widespread around the world—whether individuals have direct access to their genomic data or health-care providers and genetic counselors access and deliver it on their behalf. Not only did Brin learn he faces a higher risk of developing Parkinson's, but his situation was more serious. Why? Well, a genetic test indicating an elevated risk of disease might be interesting. But, when this information is combined with knowledge that a family member has the same condition, it is worth taking more seriously. The *combination* of Brin's ancestry and genetics suggests he is almost certain to develop Parkinson's.

Brin's brush with Medical Genealogy and his data-oriented nature prompted him to learn all he could about Parkinson's. He also modified his behavior based on studies suggesting that certain dietary and exercise choices might lower his risk of developing the disease. [103] In fact, Brin did what studies suggest many people who are confronted with concerning genetic test results do. He absorbed the information, shifted his outlook and activities, and moved on. [104] It is also worth noting that Brin's great wealth also allowed him to fund Parkinson's research, designed to improve understanding of the genetic and non-genetic components of the disease. [103]

While we are entering a new era of genetics-influenced medicine, genomics remains largely a mystery—a secretive black box that contains a combination of science and conjecture. Few understand what happens behind the scenes when DNA in spit is analyzed for a genetic test. More importantly, while genetics is advancing rapidly, there are still serious questions about whether personal genetic testing—in particular when it is used to predict the risk of disease—delivers reliable results that can be used to guide medical treatment. The U.S. Food and Drug Administration (FDA) shares this concern, which led it to send a letter to 23andMe requesting that the company stop marketing its personal genetic testing kit to consumers on November 22, 2013.[11] Understanding whether personal genomics is ready for prime time is vital—especially for those who accept the invitation of companies like 23andMe to have parts of their genome sequenced; yet, the promise of this technology and the value it could bring is undeniable. In the next part of this chapter, we'll cover some of the science and research behind the genetics revolution powering the trend we have termed Medical Genealogy.

Genome-Wide Association Studies: The Foundation of the Personal Genomics Era

Genetics is a complex science that seeks to help us answer many important questions, such as: "Where do we come from?" and "Are certain people at a higher or lower risk of disease?" In some respects, the work of geneticists can be compared to physicists who study the building blocks of matter. We used to think of atoms as the smallest particle possible. Over the decades, physicists have come to understand that atoms are made up of many sub-atomic particles that interact in different ways and, when smashed together, break up into even smaller pieces of matter.

Like atoms, scientists have learned that DNA is made up of smaller components, in this case, four proteins, or bases: adenine, cytosine, thymine, and guanine, or ACTG. These bases usually occur in pairs, A + T and C + G. DNA base pairs combine into sequences, which form DNA molecules. Sections of DNA molecules are known as genes, which influence how the body looks, functions, controls our risk for disease, and more.

Moving up the size ladder, many thousands of genes combine to form chromosomes, which also come in pairs. Normally, people have 46 (or 23 pairs) of chromosomes (half of our chromosomes come from our mothers and the other half from our fathers). A number of conditions such as Down's syndrome are caused when fetuses receive too many or too few chromosomes from their parents or they are abnormal in some way (a portion is missing, duplicated, etc.).

When investigating the genetic causes of disease, scientists started by focusing primarily on genes. Over time, they learned that differences in base pair sequences (or genetic code) can either increase the risk for, or trigger, illness. Variations in how base pairs are coded between people are called single nucleotide polymorphisms or SNPs (pronounced "snips"). SNPs are fundamental to personal genomics, so it's worth taking a little time to explain why they are important.

Take two people: Edvin and Elsa. Researchers examine their DNA and learn most of it is identical; however, they also find a small difference or mutation in a certain part of their genome. This genetic variation appears below (in bold).

Edvin (Male)
GATAGTA
CTATCAT

Elsa (Female)
GATGGTA
CTACCAT

The difference between Edvin and Elsa's DNA at the AT/GC nucleotide position shown above is what scientists refer to as a SNP. Now, SNPs in a single individual are not very meaningful. But, they become more important when found in larger groups of people. Interest in understanding the prevalence of various SNPs in many individuals led to the development of genome-wide association studies (GWAS). In GWAS-related research, scientists examine the DNA of many individuals to learn a number of things, including:

- How prevalent SNPs are within the general population or specific ethnic groups
- Whether people with different physical or mental characteristics have certain SNPs
- If those with diseases, such as Parkinson's or Alzheimer's, share SNPs

GWAS started appearing on the scientific scene around 2005 and the pace of research has sharply accelerated each year. [105] At first, scientists were excited about the potential of GWAS research to help identify the genetic causes of disease. Even more, they hoped that GWAS would help bring genetic-powered medicine to the bedside, as physicians began to use this research to guide drug and non-drug treatment, diagnose disease, and more.

So far, GWAS research has had a mixed track record. Some of the reasons for this include:

- **A Focus on More Common SNPs:** Much GWAS research has focused on SNPs that are relatively common; however, these studies have an important limitation because SNPs that are found less frequently may have a larger impact on disease. [105]

- **Limited Data on People of non-European Ancestry:** Much of the genetic material analyzed in GWAS was collected from people of European ancestry. Here's why this is a problem: At the beginning of this chapter, we talked about research suggesting that while a SNP in the ABCA7 gene was found in *both* African Americans and Caucasians, it may have a *greater influence* on the former's risk of developing Alzheimer's. Similar ethnic differences in SNP's impact are being found in other diseases such as breast cancer. [106] This suggests, in certain cases, that disease-risk assessments based on GWAS data may be less accurate when applied to non-Europeans. [107]

- **Underperforming SNPs:** This is a complex topic, but the best way to explain it may be through a hypothetical scenario. Say researchers find one (or several) SNPs thought to increase the risk of a disease, such as breast cancer. One potential next step might be to check the medical records of people with these SNPs to find out if they indeed have the condition. If there were truly a strong link between the SNP and the disease, researchers would expect to find that most people with it would have breast cancer; however, genetics is rarely this simple. Researchers have learned that many SNPs underperform. This means that some people with certain SNP profiles turn out to have diseases to which they are supposedly at risk—but many don't.

Despite these limitations, some GWAS are changing the way doctors treat patients, such as in the areas of:

- **Drug Treatment:** Researchers and pharmaceutical firms are using SNP data to help determine which patients will respond best to medications or are at higher risk of experiencing certain side effects from drugs. [105]

- **Treating Patients Before They Show Signs of a Condition:** Genetic research is beginning to help doctors identify people at risk for diabetes and heart disease earlier. One day, physicians will be able to use genetic profiling data to treat a range of illnesses before they damage the body. [105]

GWAS, SNPs and Personal Genetic Profiling

We've spent all of this time talking about GWAS and SNPs for one very import-ant reason: GWAS data powers the personal genomics industry. When people provide their DNA to companies like 23andMe, a portion of their genetic ma-terial is analyzed for the presence of SNPs. According to 23andMe's Web site:

"The technology that we use . . . analyzes approximately 1,000,000 SNPs that cover the entire genome. Although this is still only a fraction of the more than 10 million SNPs that are estimated to be in the human genome, these 1,000,000 are specially selected because they provide a lot of information about other nearby SNPs." [108]

In order to provide customers with information about their risk for disease, physi-cal characteristics (like their sense of smell and sensitivity to caffeine), 23andMe "hand-picked more than 30,000 additional SNPs of particular interest from the scientific literature." [108] Some of this literature is based on GWAS.

The personal genomics industry has attracted controversy. Some physician or-ganizations do not believe patients should have access to their genetic history without input from a doctor or genetic counselor. [104] Officials at public health agencies like the Centers for Disease Control and Prevention have warned people to "think before you spit," suggesting these tests provide little predictive power and may be inferior to a traditional method of assessing dis-ease risk: analyzing people's family history. [109] And, in late November 2013, the U.S. Food and Drug Administration asked 23andMe to stop selling its per-sonal genetic testing kits to the public.

Despite these concerns, personal genomic testing will not go away anytime soon—despite recent efforts by regulators in the United States to reign in sales of genetic testing kits to consumers. This is partly because of the widespread availability of tools that provide people with raw genetic data and the fact that genetic testing companies can operate (or deliver genetic information) in ways that do not attract regulatory scrutiny. In addition, recognizing the limits of GWAS, innovators are rapidly developing new techniques that could greatly improve our understanding of how genetics influences disease.

Where is Medical Genealogy Headed?

In mid-2013, 23andMe jump-started the direct-to-consumer genomics era by dropping the cost of their genetic screening tests to $99 and launching television advertising designed to encourage more people to take genetic tests. [110] The goal, according to 23andMe's co-founder Ann Wojcicki, is to have more than 1 million people use the service by the end of 2013. Wojcicki wants to "create a little bit of chaos" by having many people "walking around town with their genetic data." [110] While the FDA's November 2013 letter ordering the company to stop marketing its personal genetic testing kits makes it unlikely 23andMe will meet its ambitious goal, the company's marketing efforts (and controversy surrounding the FDA's letter) have significantly raised the profile of personal genetic testing.

Wojcicki, like others in the genomics arena, recognizes that genetics currently has a major data issue. While GWA studies are important, they are limited in scope, especially when it comes to providing data on people of non-European ancestry. Second, there is a need to determine the relationship between our genetic code and how genes actually influence our bodies, or phenotype. Solving these data problems will help improve understanding of the true relationship between genes and disease.

To reach the next level we need to:

• **Move from Genotyping to Sequencing:** As noted on its Website, 23and-Me does not sequence users' entire genomes. [108] Instead, the company analyzes *part* of customers' DNA to find specific SNPs. This is called genotyping. In contrast, people participating in GWAS studies have their entire DNA examined, a process known as genetic sequencing. 23andMe conducts partial DNA analysis because sequencing the entire genome is currently very expensive. Yet, having more whole genome data on larger groups of people will aid science because it will provide a much bigger pool of data for researchers to work with—especially if Asians, African Americans and other racial and ethnic groups have their genomes sequenced.

- **Examine Ancestry and Family History *in Addition* to SNPs:** Some of the most significant advances in genetics have occurred when researchers have had access to detailed information about people's family histories, ancestry and environment, in addition to their genetic profile. Combining ancestral and genetic data will only improve the methods scientists use to predict disease risk. Bringing together genetic/ancestral data also will also help people make more informed decisions about whether to take action based on a genetic test. Linking ancestral with genetic data will make Medical Genealogy more useful and widespread.

A number of technological advances in the areas of genetics, digital communication and more are combining to usher in the era of Medical Genealogy. Some of the most important developments include:

- **Whole Genome Sequencing Will Be Available for Less Than $1,000:** Traditionally, it has cost thousands of dollars to sequence a person's entire genome. However, advances in technology are making genome sequencing much cheaper. It has been long been the goal of the genomics industry to map a person's entire DNA for less than $1,000. [32] By the end of 2013, the CEO of Life Technologies Jonathan Rothberg predicts "we'll be able to do one entire human genome for $1,000." [111] And, if costs continue to drop between 50 and 90 percent over several years (as the National Institutes of Health found in 2013), we might be able to sequence people's entire genomes for hundreds of dollars by 2015. [112]
- **Social Networking-Powered Genomic Research Will Accelerate:** In addition to providing genetic testing, 23andMe enables users to share information about their family histories, diseases and more. Researchers are already tapping into 23andMe's growing data set to better understand how genes, *plus* ancestry, *plus* family history influences health. (Despite the FDA's request that 23andMe stop marketing its genetic testing kit this social networking and research activity is unlikely to cease, whether it is facilitated by 23andMe or another company.) [110]

Overall, the combination of user-generated personal data and richer genetic information may provide geneticists with the medical genealogical information they need to move beyond GWAS and gain a deeper understanding of the link between our genes, ancestry, SNPs and health.

It is important to note that the genetic revolution won't be without drawbacks. Society has not deeply considered the ethical implications of sharing and mining genetic and personal health data. Another issue is whether people — especially those with poor health and low technological literacy — will be able to process and act on medical genealogical information.

In addition, genetic counselors, physicians, public health professionals and others will be responsible for providing support and information to patients, caregivers and others struggling to understand what their genetic profiling data (augmented by information about their ancestral and family history) means and how to act on it. The issue of how best to educate the public about the benefits, drawbacks and implications of personal genetic testing came to a head when Angelina Jolie decided to undergo a double mastectomy in 2013. [113] She did this:

- Based the results of a genetic screen suggesting she had an elevated risk of breast and ovarian cancer due to a defective BRCA1 gene, and
- After considering her family history: ovarian cancer took her mother's life at the age of 56 and Jolie's aunt passed away from beast cancer in May 2013 (her aunt's genetic profile also suggested she had a high breast cancer risk) [114]

After Jolie announced her decision in a *New York Times* editorial, interest in personal genetic testing skyrocketed and a public debate was ignited about how best to use genetic information in health decision-making. [115]

So, where is the Medical Genealogy train headed? Currently, there is a great deal of uncertainty about the future of personal genetic testing in the United States given that the FDA is seeking to supervise the efforts of companies like 23andMe more closely. Will the FDA regulate the Medical Genealogy movement out of existence? We believe this is unlikely. Most importantly, as discussed above, genetic testing technologies are advancing at a rapid rate, which will likely make personal genetic data—whether interpreted by a private third-party like 23andMe, provided by physicians, or delivered in raw form—widely available. Despite the limitations of personal genetic testing and continuing questions about how best to use genomic data, Medical Genealogy has left the station and is roaring down the tracks. Regulators will continually be several steps behind efforts by innovators—whether 23andMe or other start-ups—to deliver genetic information to consumers. Moreover, Medical Genealogy is not just about personal genetic testing, but using genetic and ancestral data to develop new drugs, guide the treatment of conditions like cancer, and more. This activity is likely to accelerate as new technologies, techniques, and tools are invented and refined.

Medical Genealogy and ePatients

The personal genomics revolution is still in its infancy. However, we were curious to see how many ePatients had arranged for a genetic test to predict the risk of disease for themselves or a member of their family. This information might provide clues as to how personal genetic testing—and medical genealogy (when genetic data is linked to ancestral information)—might take shape in the future.

To answer this question, Enspektos asked ePatients participating in the 2013 edition of its digihealth pulse study the following question: Have you ever arranged a genetic test for yourself or a member of your family (before birth or afterward) to predict or understand your (or their) risk of disease? (See Appendix I for more information about digihealth pulse.)

Overall 13% of ePatients had ordered genetic testing (Figure VII). In addition:

- Among all racial groups, Asians were most likely to report having genetic testing performed
- ePatients with higher incomes (those making $76,000 per year and up) were also more likely to have arranged genetic testing than less affluent people

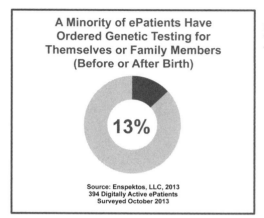

A Minority of ePatients Have Ordered Genetic Testing for Themselves or Family Members (Before or After Birth)

13%

Source: Enspektos, LLC, 2013
394 Digitally Active ePatients
Surveyed October 2013

Figure VII: Percentage of ePatients Who Arranged Genetic Testing for Themselves or a Family Member

Overall, we expect genetic testing will continue to spread as technology improves, it becomes more affordable and consumers become more aware of the benefits and drawbacks of genomic screening.

Stories: Medical Genealogy

Volunteer Labor Helps the Personal Genome Project Accelerate Genomic Research and Medical Genealogy

In 2006, Harvard geneticist George Church, one of the leaders of the Human Genome Project, identified the primary problem with using genetic data as the sole means of understanding people's health risks. He told the MIT *Technology Review's* Emily Singer: "It's hard to do genetics with just genes. You need to connect facts about the person with the facts about DNA." [116] This was the motivation for his Personal Genome Project, a global effort to advance the art and science of genetics that was founded in 2005 and has collected DNA provided by more than 2,000 volunteers as of 2012. [117]

At its core, the Personal Genome Project is an ideal representation of Medical Genealogy: combining genetic material with information about people's family, medical and nutrition histories. According to its Website, the Personal Genome Project aims to accelerate genetic research by developing "a collection of many human genomes that remain connected to their owners who contribute additional information over their lifetime." Because of the possibility people participating in the project may be identified (via their genome) at a later date, they must complete a rigorous application process designed to ensure they understand the consequences of publicly sharing their DNA.

Learn More: http://www.personalgenomes.org

Molecular Autopsies: Using the Genetic Material of the Dead to Aid the Living

Fueled by demand from concerned family members of young people with unexplained "mystery deaths," genetic tests are being performed on the recently deceased in an effort to uncover potentially deadly rare heart conditions or other medical problems that may be genetic in origin and affect other family members. The intent is to use test results to help living family members understand their risk for disease and potentially save lives.

Learn More:

http://www.mercurynews.com/science/ci_17314134

http://www.ncbi.nlm.nih.gov/pubmed/22677073

---

[10] Common genetic variations or mutations among people are called single nucleotide polymorphisms, or SNPs. Most SNPs have no influence on our health, but a few may predict how people respond to drugs, react to harmful environmental chemicals, or suggest a person has a higher risk of developing certain diseases. You'll learn more about SNPs later in this chapter.

[11] To view the FDA's letter to 23andMe, please visit http://www.fda.gov/ICECI/EnforcementActions/WarningLetters/2013/ucm376296.htm

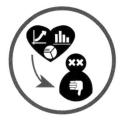

Trend 6:
The Over-Quantified Self

As the volume of clinical and health data increases (collected from wearable computers, passive sensors, and more), consumers will struggle to make sense of the flood of information they produce. Some may ignore this data; others might look for ways to simplify it using technology, while the rest will turn to trusted medical intermediaries for assistance and advice.

In 2001, UNICEF's Innocenti Research Centre issued a shocking report on the rate of child deaths in 26 of the world's wealthiest nations. [118] The Centre estimated that nearly 20,000 children in rich countries would die from injuries during the next twelve months. Which nation was at the top of what the Centre called its "Child Injury Death League?" South Korea. UNICEF reported that nearly 13,000 Korean children between the ages of 1 and 14 had died due to injuries between 1991 and 1995. [118]

Why were so many young children dying in South Korea? The Centre concluded that cars were to blame. But many of the children being killed were not riding in vehicles; instead, cars were hitting them while they were walking in the street. Korean officials immediately took a number of steps to protect children from cars including passing legislation requiring lower speed limits on roads and funding the placement of traffic control devices such as speed bumps near schools.

Unfortunately, none of these tactics managed to effectively decrease the rate of child traffic fatalities. In fact, statistics suggested that accidents occurring near schools actually *increased* after the legislation was passed. [119] If drivers were ignoring the law and road features designed to calm school-area traffic, what would convince them to slow down?

Finally in desperation, Korean traffic officials uncovered the behavioral insight that providing people with real-time information about how fast they were driving might be an ideal way to get them to stop speeding. In a pilot project, they placed electronic signs displaying data on drivers' speed on several roads near schools. It worked. In fact, the results were so pronounced, this tactic has been copied around the world.

It's likely that you've seen these speed-monitoring displays, or SMDs, in your travels. SMDs generally display two pieces of information:

- The area speed limit, e.g., 20 mph
- The speed of the car, e.g., 35 mph

These SMDs succeeded where legislation failed. [120] On average, Koreans drove 18 percent slower shortly after SMDs were installed. And, these speed reductions persisted over the long term. While average speeds crept up over time, people still drove an average of 12 percent slower than before SMDs were placed on roads near schools. [119]

Influencing Human Behavior Using Data: Feedback Loops, Libertarian Paternalism, and the Quantified Self

This tale of speeding South Koreans illustrates how data-powered behavioral feedback loops can be used to nudge people to act in different ways. In this case, drivers were provided with real-time information about whether their behavior (driving speed) was acceptable. Many speeding drivers—perhaps in-stinctively—chose to slow down when confronted with information indicating they were being watched and their actions were putting the lives of school children in danger.

Data has taken center stage in the battle to encourage people to act in ways that benefit their health such as quitting smoking, exercising more, and eating healthfully. [120] At the level of countries and governments, data from studies examining human behavior is being used to develop a range of health-related policies. For example, the United Kingdom's Behavioural Insights Team (or "Nudge Unit") has initiated data-informed public health projects designed to spur organ donation, reduce teen pregnancies, and more. [121] This form of what Richard Thaler and Cass Sunstein refer to as **"libertarian paternalism"** has also taken root in the United States. [122] In fact, Sunstein formerly ran the U.S. Office of Information and Regulatory Affairs where he used behavioral data to refine and craft a range of federal policies and regulations. [123]

At the individual level, the idea that data—particularly if it is collected on a regular basis over a long period of time—can be used to change behavior (es-pecially in the area of health) is also at the core of what has come to be known as the quantified self-movement. Melanie Swan of the MS Futures Group has described quantified self as "the act of individuals self-tracking any kind of bio-logical, physical, behavioral, or environmental information." [124]

How widespread is health tracking? In 2013, the Pew Research Center report-ed that 69% of Americans tracked some form of "health indicator for them-selves or a loved one;" however, most Americans are not using digital tools such as mobile apps to self-track. [125] Pew found that only 21% "use some form of technology to track their health data." In the 2013 edition of its digihealth pulse study, Enspektos found that 39% of ePatients use Web sites, mobile apps, or other digital tools to track their health data.

Quantified self-enthusiasts suggest that the act of collecting and monitoring health data has numerous benefits. Most importantly, they believe that peo-ple who receive instant feedback on the results of their health actions (such as reduced resting-heart rate after exercise or weight loss) will ultimately be healthier. There is some evidence to support this argument. Pew found that self-trackers who record their health data using technology or written notes are more likely to say doing so has helped them interact with doctors or changed "their overall approach to health." [125] In addition, "quantified selfers" have offered anecdotal evidence that health self-tracking has enabled them to lose weight, kept them motivated to exercise, and more.

Traditionally, health self-tracking has required a large time commitment. People have had to manually enter health data into a Web- or computer-based database, juggle multiple devices, and be disciplined about collecting, analyzing, and taking action on data.

As we'll discuss below, these problems are far from solved; however, new technologies such as mobile phones, watches, and bracelets are making it easier for people to self-track. In fact, self-tracking tools that require less work may also do a better job of helping people improve their health. For example, a study published in the *Journal of Medical Internet Research* in 2013 comparing the benefits of self-tracking using smartphones, Web sites, and written diaries indicates that those using mobile devices to self-track lost more weight and continued tracking for a longer period of time. [126]

Although many people are not currently using technology to track their health statuses, there are signs that the quantified self-movement may become more popular over the next few years. While most people won't think of themselves as quantified selfers, wearable devices like fitness bands and watches may reach a broad audience. For example, analysts at Business Intelligence predict that more than 100 million wearable devices will be sold worldwide by 2014. [127]

The growing popularity of self-tracking devices (like wearables) and a growing belief in the power of data to change health behavior will impact patients, caregivers, and others in profound ways. Most importantly, these trends will help to accelerate the personalized health movement, as people will have access to vast amounts of information about themselves and their families; moreover, businesses, government, insurers, and others will increasingly ask consumers to collect their health data and take action based on what they learn.

It is worth taking a step back to ask whether there is a downside to the quantified self-movement. Will having more health data actually improve health? Are technology and device developers spending enough time thinking about whether people will be able to understand and act on the data they receive? Liam Ryan, CEO of GetHealth, an Ireland-based company that has produced a wellness-related mobile and online application, believes the answer is no. In a provocative October 2013 blog post, he wrote, "Nowhere do [sensing] devices tell you how to improve your numbers, or what numbers are most worth improving. You are left with a screen full of detailed metrics with peaks and troughs, but no straight-forward, clear advice on what are the best ways to improve these magical numbers." [128] The disconnect Ryan identified between the delivery of health data and consumers' ability to take action on this information is part of a trend we have coined the Over-Quantified Self.

The Over-Quantified Self: When Consumers Resist or Reject Health Self-Tracking

It wouldn't be a stretch to suggest that those within the quantified self-movement (and their allies in health organizations, startups, and government) are part of a technology-powered health subculture. Like people in all cultures, quantified selfers share a set of values and assumptions about the world. Although she didn't limit her analysis to the quantified self-movement, Deborah Lupton, a professor of sociology at the University of Sydney, described some of these shared beliefs in a 2013 article published in the journal *Social Theory and Health*, including: [129]

- **Digital Technologies Are The Best Way for Empowered Patients to Control Their Bodies:** In some respects, health can be viewed as a struggle for control over our bodies. Quantified selfers believe that by using technological devices to monitor their bodily functions (and dysfunctions), patients can become truly empowered and have a greater measure of control over their health. Some also think that everyone should be able to make sense of their health data and juggle the multiple devices required to collect and manage this information.

- **The Home, Not the Clinic, Should Be the Center of Care:** In an environment where patients have access to sophisticated health information via sensing devices, there is less need for them to travel to clinics, hospitals, and other traditional centers of care. With health data and communications technologies, doctors can virtually deliver care wherever the patient happens to be. Some quantified selfers welcome the rise of the home as the center of care and the shift in the balance of power from health provider to patient. [130]
- **Because People Are Undisciplined and Unmotivated About Their Health, Digital Surveillance Technologies Are Needed to Keep Them in Line:** Lupton has noted that there is a disciplinary component to self-tracking and surveillance technologies. In addition to being monitored, patients are prodded with reminders to take their medications and engage with others around their care. Some quantified selfers may welcome the fact that digital health tools can motivate and discipline patients—especially those they feel are not doing enough to maintain their health.

Some patients and caregivers may have no problem accepting these assumptions and acting in ways that are culturally acceptable to quantified selfers; however, others may not. The *over-quantified self* becomes a problem when people are asked or required to collect and use health data in ways they are unwilling or unable to. Consequences of the over-quantified self include:

- **Information Overload:** Some patients may be unable to use the vast amounts of data provided by sensors and other devices to improve their health
- **Device Frustration:** People may be frustrated when asked to use multiple technologies to track their health—especially when devices fail to communicate or share data with each other
- **Resentment:** Some consumers may resent being constantly reminded to manage their health in certain ways (e.g., exercise or take medications) when using self-tracking devices

Jody Ranck is a digital health futurist and author of *Connected Health: How Mobile Phones, Cloud and Big Data Will Reinvent Healthcare*. He has also been a longtime user of self-tracking technologies for fitness purposes. Ranck is concerned about assumptions that people will be able to make sense of large amounts of sophisticated health data and be willing to manage it using multiple devices. In an interview conducted for this book, Ranck made a number of observations about the quantified self-movement, including:

- **We Can't Assume People Will Self-Track Over the Long-Term:** "The assumption [that people are willing and able to self-track] has very little evidence to support it and is more of a marketing 'Hail Mary' than reality. In fact, many people who are not . . . relatively healthy white males . . . but are suffering from chronic diseases actually get quite sick of quantification."
- **Quantified Self Must Prove its Worth:** "If we look closely at segments [where health spending is highest] such as the poor, I'm willing to bet that trackers, as we know them, will not be popular [in these groups]. Yet it is among the poor and people with chronic conditions where we need to move the dial on outcomes if we are to prove the worthiness of digital health."
- **We Need to Help People Take Action on Their Health Data:** "We know, for example, that few tracking devices can communicate with electronic medical records currently. It's all well and good to track things, but if there is no service that can provide thoughtful feedback and guidance, then the energy put into tracking can be cumbersome for very little gain. I'm waiting to see the products and services that provide feedback/support (based on health data) that shifts outcomes in a measurable way before I jump on the quantified self bandwagon."

Are ePatients Concerned About the Over-Quantified Self?

It's one thing for digital health technology developers and experts to be concerned about the over-quantified self, but what about ePatients? To find out, Enspektos asked ePatients participating in the 2013 edition of its digihealth pulse study whether they were worried that using health self-tracking devices could lead to information overload. ePatients were told that companies have developed devices that can provide a lot of information about their personal health (daily, hourly, and weekly). They were then asked to rate their level of concern about whether these tools could provide them with too much health information using a scale from 1 to 5 (1 = low concern; 3 = moderate concern; 5 = very high concern).

Overall, more than half of ePatients (57%) said they had moderate-to-high levels of concern that health self-tracking devices could deliver too much information (Figure VIII).[12] Interestingly, people with chronic conditions (such as high blood pressure and cancer) were less concerned about information overload than ePatients without them (Figure IX). This may be because ePatients with chronic conditions might welcome receiving detailed information about their health on a regular basis, as this data could help them better manage their care.

On the other hand, people without chronic conditions are the primary audience for many companies selling self-tracking technologies for fitness and other purposes. Health organizations developing, marketing, or deploying these technologies should pay close attention to ePatients' concerns that using these devices could lead to health-data overload.

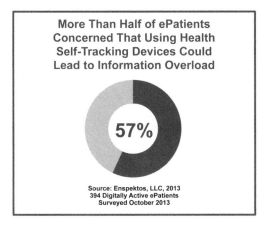

More Than Half of ePatients Concerned That Using Health Self-Tracking Devices Could Lead to Information Overload

57%

Source: Enspektos, LLC, 2013
394 Digitally Active ePatients
Surveyed October 2013

Figure VIII: Percentage of ePatients Having Moderate to Very High Concern Using Health Self-Tracking Devices Could Lead to Information Overload

Figure IX: Percentage of ePatients With and Without Chronic Conditions Moderately to Very Highly Concerned That Using Health Self-Tracking Devices Could Lead to Information Overload

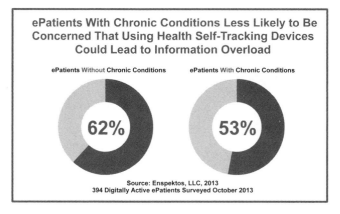

ePatients With Chronic Conditions Less Likely to Be Concerned That Using Health Self-Tracking Devices Could Lead to Information Overload

ePatients Without Chronic Conditions ePatients With Chronic Conditions

62% 53%

Source: Enspektos, LLC, 2013
394 Digitally Active ePatients Surveyed October 2013

Stories: Fostering and Fighting the Over-Quantified Self

Withings Health Cloud: Much Data, But Less Actionable Information

One of the most prominent leaders in the quantified self space is health-care technology company Withings. With an array of products ranging from movement trackers to wireless body scales, the company's range of tools allows for multiple types of tracking and data collection.

More than any other company, they have also taken a page from Apple's book and worked to foster an ecosystem that can add more functionality to their products. Calling it the "Health Cloud," this platform brings together over 100 tracking apps from multiple systems that all integrate and use data from Withings' products. The result is a myriad of opportunities for consumers to integrate with any tracking service to capture as much data as they can—without necessarily being able to integrate or act on that data.

Learn More: http://blog.withings.com/en/2013/05/30/super-charge-your-withings-experience-with-100-partner-apps-and-ifttt/

Qualcomm Wireless Reach: Working With Doctors to Avoid the Over-Quantified Self

One of the rare stories of a company using quantified self-data to move beyond the confusion is Qualcomm. The brand has launched a program called Wireless Reach in China that uses electrocardiogram-sensing handsets to capture 30 seconds of heart data and transmit that information electronically to a 24-hour service center in Beijing. Most importantly, to avoid the over-quantification trap, the center where this data is sent actually has more than 40 physicians on call to provide a remote diagnosis to patients in underserved areas and give real-time advice to those with cardiovascular diseases.

Learn More:

http://www.insidepolitics.org/brookingsreports/mobile_health_52212.pdf

---

[12] Percentage of ePatients rating level of concern as 3 (moderate), 4 (high), and 5 (very high) is shown in Figures VIII and IX.

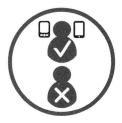

Trend 7:
The Device Divide

Today, the "digital divide" separates those who can access the latest digital tools from those who cannot. In digital health, we face a "Device Divide." This refers to the fact that economic disparities may prevent patients, providers, hospitals, and clinics from accessing the latest technological innovations.

Don Jones, who serves as vice president of global strategy and market development at Qualcomm Life, has a big problem with most digital health startups: they think too small. Speaking at the 2012 Digital Health Summer Summit, Jones talked about how many products are not optimized to solve health's biggest problems because they are focused on addressing a single issue in consumers' lives. For example, it is always helpful for patients to receive reminders about whether to take their medications; however, it would be more useful and impactful if a product were to help them manage every aspect of their prescription drug needs, including understanding the potential side effects associated with taking multiple medications. [131]

One of the biggest problems in health care today is the rising rate of chronic conditions such as diabetes, depression, and heart disease. Chronic illnesses exact a tremendous toll as the leading cause of sickness and death globally; moreover, chronic diseases account for nearly 85% of health spending in the United States. [132] In 2011, the World Economic Forum released its first study on the total global costs of non-communicable diseases and concluded that, on a worldwide level, "the cumulative costs of CVD, chronic respiratory disease, cancer, and diabetes in low- and middle-income countries are estimated to surpass USD 7 trillion in 2011-2025, an average of nearly USD 500 billion per year." [133]

While chronic conditions are a serious issue globally, they are especially problematic for seniors, ethnic and racial minorities, and the poor in the United States. [132] About half of men and women over 65 have two or more chronic diseases. [132] Minorities are especially likely to have some conditions such as diabetes. [134] People earning less money tend to have more excess body fat and higher rates of obesity than higher-income individuals. [135]

Digital health technologies have the potential to reduce the prevalence and impact of chronic conditions. But, their benefits will be blunted if people from underserved populations and the health providers serving them don't have access to these innovations. If not aggressively addressed, the device divide is a significant issue that has the potential to worsen over the next few years as the use of health technologies expands.

Both Providers and Patients Face the Device Divide

When thinking about technological divides, it is easy to see it solely in terms of access to treatments or devices for patients. The truth is, it is vital to ask if physicians, nurses, and others have equal access to the latest innovations and technologies as well.

One particularly concerning area that has received a lot of attention over the past several years is the slow adoption of electronic health records (EHRs) in some clinics, hospitals, and other facilities located in underserved areas of the U.S. Over the past few years, fueled by government financial incentives, health organizations, physicians, and others have been racing to purchase and implement systems to use EHRs. Despite this, communities with higher percentages of minority and low-income populations are far less likely to have EHRs in place. [136]

Ironically, EHRs may be even more important for these underserved populations as compared to other groups. For example, many low-income patients switch doctors frequently due to economic or other reasons. In some cases, these individuals have had to carry paper records from physician to physician when changing providers. EHRs can ensure patients and their doctors have access to a single accurate and complete health record.

In addition, EHRs can also have significant public health benefits, including aiding the collection of important data on disease rates, quality, medications, and more. (See our discussion of the predictive psychohistory trend for more information about these benefits.) Information collection is especially important because it has traditionally been difficult to gather accurate and complete data on issues related to health disparities and quality of care in underserved communities. [137]

Fortunately, some are taking steps to address the EHR access problem. Widely considered one of the global leaders in the national adoption of EHRs, Singapore's Nationwide Electronic Health Record system (NEHR) and its "one patient, one record" vision is viewed as a pioneering effort in the EHR field. [138] Building upon its natural advantage as a relatively small nation of geographically concentrated citizens, Singapore's EHR model works across all levels of the population. Even in the dramatically more complex United States, the U.S. government has responded to the provider device divide by implementing initiatives designed to ensure facilities serving people living in low-income, rural, and minority communities can purchase EHRs. [136]

All of this points to some positive news about addressing this divide on the provider side, as governments are working to address the issue. But, what about the patients?

Happily, there are signs that the digital divide (poor access to digital tools such as computers and the Web in certain groups) may be narrowing for patients as well. Here's one powerful example. Disparities in home-based Internet access have traditionally been an issue in low-income and minority communities. Today, the rising popularity of cell and smartphones has made Internet and computer access less of a problem. For example, according to a 2013 report published by the Pew Research Center, "young adults, non-whites, and those with relatively low income and educational levels [were more likely to rely solely] on their cell phones to access the Web." [139]

Looking at health, it is clear that minorities and the poor have not been left behind by the technology revolution. In the digihealth pulse research conducted in September 2012, Enspektos found that among low-income U.S. ePatients (those making less than $30,000 annually):[13]

- Thirty-seven percent used the mobile Web frequently or very frequently to search for health information
- One-third of mobile users had downloaded health apps to their devices

While mobile device access has reduced some aspects of the device divide for underserved groups, it has not solved others. For example:

- Some health technologies require the use of a home computer and high-speed Internet access, which low-income Americans are less likely to possess.
- Although people may own mobile devices, they may be unable to use health applications that require information to be constantly uploaded and downloaded due to caps their plans place on data access.
- Device manufacturers like Apple are constantly rolling out software and hardware upgrades. Although carriers subsidize the cost of devices, accessing a new mobile phone sometimes requires signing up for a lengthy and expensive contract. This may limit the reach of certain health applications that require new devices and software to operate.

The final element of this patient-side device divide to consider is related to the actual technology and devices themselves. According to global information company IHS, the world market for consumer medical devices is poised to grow dramatically in coming years. In 2013, global revenue from sales of medical devices grew by 4% to a robust $8.2 billion. By 2017, device revenue is projected to grow to $10.6 billion. [140]

A key source for this growth will be the country of Israel, where there are projected to be more than 700 medical device companies as of August 2013. Espicom Business Intelligence estimates that the Israeli market for medical devices alone will top $1 billion by 2016. [141] Given the emerging demand from the world's two largest nations—India and China—Israel is perfectly poised to serve the demand from both of those markets.

But why is the medical devices industry growing so quickly? One reason is the globally aging population that will require more devices such as hip and knee replacements to combat the most common age-related injuries. Another is the increasing number of people worldwide who are managing chronic conditions at a younger and younger age, those who will require devices such as blood glucose meters or blood pressure monitors.

A side effect of the growth in demand for medical devices is that costs are rising dramatically as well. Cutting edge prosthetic devices can run hundreds of thousands of dollars, for example, putting them far out of reach for those who are not independently wealthy or in possession of unbelievably generous insurance plans.

On many levels, this is creating a *functional* device divide as it applies to access to medical devices that carry hefty price tags, which no one but the most privileged will be able to afford.

ePatients and the Device Divide: Is it About Optional Versus Essential Health Technology?

Enspektos examined the question of access in the 2013 edition of its digihealth pulse study by looking at whether ePatients reported having trouble accessing or purchasing health technology innovations (such as mobile health apps, wearable devices like Fitbit, and Web sites) due to financial considerations.

Enspektos found that among ePatients who wanted to purchase/access health tech, 42% said financial considerations prevented them from doing so (Figure X). In addition, people from across income groups (affluent to poor) cited financial concerns as a barrier to access.

One question to ask about this data is why the percentage of ePatients who say financial reasons prevented them from accessing or purchasing health technology is so high. Enspektos believes part of the reason may be how people make decisions about items they want versus need. For example, a more affluent ePatient may want to have the latest wearable fitness device, but decide not to purchase it because it isn't essential.

For people making less money the decision-making process may be different. These individuals might be unable to purchase (or access) a more expensive innovation because they lack access to high speed Internet, a smartphone, or a high volume mobile data plan.

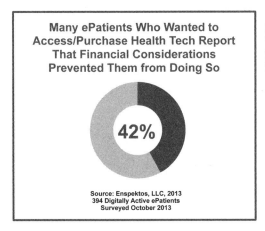

Many ePatients Who Wanted to Access/Purchase Health Tech Report That Financial Considerations Prevented Them from Doing So

42%

Source: Enspektos, LLC, 2013
394 Digitally Active ePatients
Surveyed October 2013

Figure X: Percentage of ePatients Who Report Wanting to Purchase/ Access Health Technology But Cited Financial Considerations As a Reason They Did Not

When looking at the device divide question from a race perspective, Enspektos found something surprising. More than half of African American ePatients said financial considerations prevented them from accessing health tech versus just over one-third of whites (Figure XI). African Americans and whites from a range of income groups (poor to affluent) cited financial reasons as a barrier to access.

Figure XI: Percentage of ePatients Who Report Wanting to Purchase/Access Health Technology But Cited Financial Considerations As a Reason They Did Not (By Race)

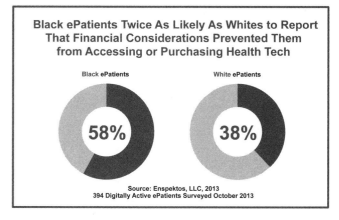

In future editions of digihealth pulse, Enspektos plans to look at the device divide question further—specifically, whether people who view health technologies as essential have not been able to access them because of financial considerations.

Stories: Combating the Device Divide Around the World

A number of organizations, public-private partnerships, and others have launched initiatives and products designed to broaden access to health technology and device innovations. Some stories related to these efforts appear below.

UCL Institute of Health Equity: Reducing Disparities in Medical Care, Technology Access, and Beyond

In November of 2011, the Institute of Health Equity (IHE) was born from research completed by University College London Professor Sir Michael Marmot and his team of investigators. Supported by several UK based organizations, the IHE focuses on conducting research and shining a spotlight on health-care inequities across the globe. To affect change, the IHE focuses on influencing global and local policies, learning and sharing best practices, identifying research gaps to build an evidence base, and training or mentoring. Perhaps most importantly, the organization is one of the global leaders in bringing more attention, research, and political pressure around the inequity in health that has led to what we have called the device divide.

Learn More: http://www.instituteofhealthequity.org/about

Dorset Orthopaedic Delivers Innovations in Prosthetics, But at a High Cost

In December 2008, a week-old baby named Marshall Janson was rushed to the hospital following an attack of meningococcal meningitis. Doctors were able to save young Marshall's life, but his hands and legs had to be amputated. His family, wanting to give the boy a chance at a normal life, visited prosthetic limb maker Dorset Orthopaedic to have him fitted for a pair of $20,000 prosthetic blades (the same style popularized by controversial Paralympic athlete Oscar Pistorius). The family, hoping to support the financial costs of fitting Marshall with additional prosthetics as he grows up, created a charity called "The HANDSTAND Appeal" to raise the nearly $1.5 million it is anticipated these devices will cost throughout Marshall's life. The story is a perfect example of the device divide as it relates to the spread of medical technology. Innovative companies like Dorset are pioneering solutions, but the high costs make them only available today to a limited market of the privileged or those with the means and ability to solicit donations. With the costs of most new prosthetic limbs ranging between $5,000 and upwards of $50,000, the most innovative solutions may be out of reach for those with limited ability to pay for them.

Learn More:

http://www.dorset-ortho.com/prosthetics/prosthetic-limbs/

http://www.handstand.org.uk/

ColaLife: Using a Soft Drink Maker's Global Reach to Deliver Medical Innovations to the Underserved

One of the biggest problems in developing countries is the rate of mortality among young children. One in eight children die before their fifth birthday and the second biggest killer isn't some exotic disease—it is diarrhea. These deaths could be easily prevented with the right treatments, yet medicine is notoriously difficult to transport to rural areas. There is one organization, though, that has cracked the code on how to reach people living in even the most remote locations: Coca-Cola. So several years ago this basic fact led to an innovative thought: what if vaccine makers could piggyback on Coca-Cola's vast distribution network? Thus ColaLife was born. Through specialized anti-diarrhea kits (Kit Yamoyo) that fit in the spaces between crates of Coca-Cola bottles, the ColaLife team has developed an award-winning solution to a common problem—and addressed the third world device divide problem (related to access to tools and technologies that deliver medical treatments to rural areas) in an important and sustainable way.

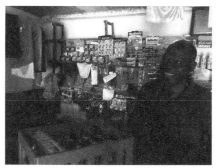

A Kit Yamoyo retailer in Katete talks about his experiences selling the anti-diarrheal kit to mothers. At the bottom of the image, two Kit Yamoyos rest in the empty spaces between crated bottles.

Photo Credit: Rohit Ramachandani, ColaLife

---

[13] See Appendix I for more information about digihealth pulse.

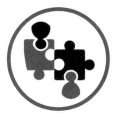

Trend 8:
Multicultural Misalignment

*Digital health technologies will be less effective if they are not opti-
mized, or personalized, to account for differences in gender, age, culture,
ethnicity, knowledge, literacy, and more. Multicultural misalignment
refers to the problems caused by applying standardized or generic technology solutions to diverse populations. A number of organizations and
businesses will address this issue in innovative and effective ways.*

Does the digital technology industry have a diversity problem?

In 2011, this was the question of the moment after a documentary, *Black in
America: The New Promised Land: Silicon Valley*, first aired on CNN. Founder
of *TechCrunch* and influential blogger Michael Arrington, who was featured in
the broadcast, appeared to confirm perceptions of Silicon Valley as unfriendly
to minorities. When asked if he knew any African American entrepreneurs he
replied: "I don't know a single [one]." [142]

Arrington later recanted his statement, saying he was surprised by the question and indeed knew many African American technology founders. [143] Although Arrington accused Soledad O'Brien, who conducted the interview, of

being dishonest, CNN did succeed in its goal: to raise serious questions about whether African Americans, Hispanics, women, and other groups are well-represented in the innovation economy.

While the controversy ignited by *Black in America* has cooled, the documentary has had far-reaching effects. Most notably, Hank Williams, a well-regarded black technology entrepreneur, who was profiled in the documentary, was inspired to embark on a quest to address the structural, economic, and societal barriers facing women, African Americans, and others seeking to launch and grow digital startups. As part of this effort, Williams launched *Platform*, a non-profit designed to "increase the interest, participation, and success of those under-represented in the innovation economy." In June 2013, Williams organized Platform's first conference, which attracted participation from a range of luminaries, including Massachusetts Governor Deval Patrick and General Colin Powell.

But Williams' quest isn't about diversity for diversity's sake. Rather, he believes diversifying digital is an urgent economic issue. Writing in the *Huffington Post*, Williams argued: "The endless flood of location-aware/social/e-commerce apps certainly suggests that we need fresh ideas from outside the current technology monoculture." He continued: "It isn't news that a monoculture precludes a diversity of thought and creates an inbred ecosystem." His conclusion is well-founded in research. Williams cited "two prestigious European institutions," that have "published studies showing that not only do diverse teams create unique ideas, but they result in a more productive workplace." [144]

If seeking out and fostering diverse perspectives is critical in the innovation economy, it is worth asking in this discussion of our multicultural misalignment trend if the health industry itself has a diversity problem. For some, the answer is a clear "yes."

The Health Industry Diversity Gap

In 2012, Rock Health published a report called Women in Health, which focused on the gender gap in health-care leadership positions. Although women make up 73% of "medical and health services managers and 47% of medical school graduates," only 4% (a noticeably low number) are CEOs of health-care companies. [145]

Do the gender disparities Rock Health identified extend to health technology companies and digital health startups? "Absolutely," asserted noted digital health analyst and business development consultant, Bonnie Feldman in an interview conducted for this book. "There are very few women in leadership positions in health technology despite the fact that they really drive the health decisions of their families."

In the previous chapter we focused on how people from underserved communities (such as low-income women, African Americans, and Hispanics) tend to be more likely to suffer from certain chronic conditions that are driving health spending in the U.S. Given the importance of reducing disease and improving the wellbeing of people from these groups, it's vital that they be well served by the health technology sector. Are digital health innovators paying enough attention to the needs of people from these groups?

"At this point, I would say no," Andre Blackman, founder of the digital communications consultancy Pulse + Signal and respected health innovation evangelist told us. He suggests that part of the problem is the perception that people from underserved communities are not using digital technologies. On the contrary he argues, "[people from these groups] are early adopters and are quite interested in using innovative tools for important things like managing their health."

Dr. Ivor Braden Horn, a physician with a special passion for bringing health technologies to underserved populations, believes another issue is the lack of a dedicated "ecosystem that promotes the development, implementation, and evaluation of . . . technology solutions geared toward minority populations who need it the most." [146] However, she believes things are slowly changing as more people recognize the importance of bringing people from diverse backgrounds and perspectives into the health innovation economy. [146]

Gender and ethnic under-representation are not the only causes for concern. Feldman also highlighted the issue of age. Currently, increasing numbers of middle-aged people are coping with their own health issues while caring for aging parents. Despite this, Feldman has noticed that "almost no one in the middle" is leading many digital health startups. "The age gap is as shocking as gender disparities in the health technology ecosystem," Feldman told us.

The Connection Between Multicultural Misalignment and Poor User Engagement With Health Technologies

Lack of diversity has the potential to greatly diminish technology's ability to solve the biggest problems in health. Perhaps the most important threat health innovators face is lack of user engagement with the tools they develop. Simply put, if people from diverse communities don't use digital health technologies, this tech will fail at shaping and encouraging positive health behaviors; unfortunately, there is evidence that health technology developers have not thought enough about the role culture, technological literacy, economics, and other factors that play in accelerating or blunting user engagement—especially among the underserved.

In 2008, the U.S. Agency for Healthcare Research and Quality published an extensive report examining some of the obstacles to greater health technology use among the elderly, underserved, and chronically ill. [147] The authors of the report identified a number of issues (based on an extensive analysis of previous research) contributing to low user engagement with health technology solutions that are still relevant today (and will continue to be tomorrow) including:

- **Lack of Technological Literacy:** In some cases, low-income people were unable to use certain technologies because they had limited experience with computers. This is a prime example of the Participation Gap, or disparities in people's ability to efficiently use technology caused by limited exposure to digital tools. [148]
- **Poor Usability:** At times, technology users found certain tools difficult to use (e.g., poor button color or placement) or that content was written in overly technical language.

- **A Belief That Solutions Were of Limited Benefit:** When choosing to stop using a tool, some said they had little confidence the technology could help them as a major reason for their decision. This was especially true in cases where tools required users to enter large amounts of data on a regular basis.

- **Tools Did Not Fit Into Users' Lifestyles:** Another major reason for poor user engagement was that people found it hard to fit tools into their day-to-day lives—e.g., when people are asked to regularly log health data using the Web, but don't have Internet access at home.

- **Messages Were Not Believable:** Tools that delivered information that contradicted users' personal experiences tended to do poorly (for example, asthma patients received an alert from a computerized system asking them to increase their medication dosage but many ignored this message because they were never asked to do this in the past). In addition, when the rationale for recommended health actions was not explained, people were less apt to follow them. [149]

The factors contributing to poor user engagement listed above apply to people of all ethnic, cultural, and age groups; however, the issues of trust, usability, literacy, and whether technology fits into people's lifestyles may be especially relevant to seniors and people from underserved communities. If they cannot view the world through the eyes of women, diverse and low-income populations, it can be hard for technology developers to anticipate and appropriately respond to these issues.

The problems caused by developers' lack of understanding of issues important to diverse populations were highlighted during the 2013 MedCity News CONVERGE conference as well. Event organizers invited 50 local members of the Philadelphia AARP Chapter to CONVERGE where they offered their perspective to health technology entrepreneurs participating in the Pfizer Startup Showcase. [150] Some of the feedback AARP members provided to entrepreneurs include:

- **Don't Forget Health Care's Social Component:** Some seniors were not persuaded by entrepreneurs' arguments that technology could help them become more efficient. For them a doctor's visit is a social event where they have an opportunity to leave their homes and interact with others. Taking the time to socialize with physicians and others before and during a doctor's appointment was more important than being efficient.

- **Build Tools That Add Value to Our Lives:** Seniors were less focused on functionality than value—specifically how these tools could help them improve or understand their health.

At the end of the day, preventing multicultural misalignment is all about ensuring health innovations *benefit all* segments of society. In our discussion, Blackman offered this warning, "If digital health innovators only direct products and services toward limited parts of the population, over time technology will stagnate rather than advance."

Multicultural Misalignment and ePatients

As discussed above, ensuring that consumer-facing health technologies are culturally appropriate and fit within people's lifestyles is vitally important; yet, do ePatients who have used digital health technologies agree?

Enspektos addressed this issue in the 2013 edition of its digihealth pulse study.[14] ePatients were asked to think about the last time they used a health-related technology such as a Web site, mobile health application, or something else. ePatients were then asked to rate how important (i.e., not important, important, or very important) it was that the tech:

- Fit within their lifestyles
- Reflected or matched their background/culture/preferences, etc.

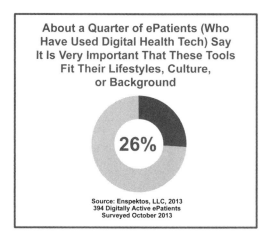

About a Quarter of ePatients (Who Have Used Digital Health Tech) Say It Is Very Important That These Tools Fit Their Lifestyles, Culture, or Background

Figure XII: Percentage of ePatients Who Say Culturally/Background/Lifestyle Appropriate Digital Health Tech is Very Important

26%

Source: Enspektos, LLC, 2013
394 Digitally Active ePatients
Surveyed October 2013

Figure XIII: Percentage of ePatients Who Say Culturally/Background/Lifestyle Appropriate Digital Health Tech is Very Important (By Race)

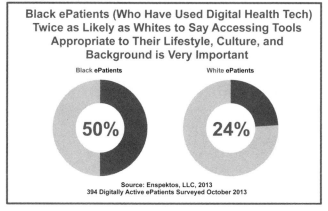

Black ePatients (Who Have Used Digital Health Tech) Twice as Likely as Whites to Say Accessing Tools Appropriate to Their Lifestyle, Culture, and Background is Very Important

Black ePatients · White ePatients

50% · 24%

Source: Enspektos, LLC, 2013
394 Digitally Active ePatients Surveyed October 2013

Overall (among those who had used digital health tech), 26% said it was very important that these tools fit their lifestyles, culture, or background (Figure XII).

Enspektos did not find large differences between groups on this question from an income or age perspective; however, African American ePatients were twice as likely as whites to say using lifestyle or background/culturally appropriate tech was very important (Figure XIII).

This research suggests that health technology innovators, developers, and others should think carefully about how to develop tools that fit the needs, culture, and background of all groups. Here are a few stories of organizations and people addressing this issue.

Stories: Multicultural Misalignment

"Carmen" The Virtual Advisor Inspires Low-Income Adults to Walk More

One of the biggest problems in underserved communities and particularly among the elderly is a lack of physical activity. This leads to many other health problems, and tends to be an extremely difficult challenge to solve. In 2011, Stanford University Professor of Health Research & Policy and Medicine, Dr. Abby King presented the results of a pilot test program using a virtual Hispanic advisor named "Carmen" (who also spoke Spanish) to help motivate and engage low-income ethnic minority older adults (over 55) living in San Jose, CA. People who interacted with Carmen ultimately walked five times longer than those who didn't (based on measurements taken with a pedometer. Six out of seven participants also reported they "felt close" to and "trusted" Carmen, and 95% of the participants accessed her program after the study ended.

Learn More:

http://www.slideshare.net/PersuasiveTechLab/mobile-health2011-slide-skingfinal

Avoiding the Percentile Chart Trap

A first-time parent can find an excuse to panic about almost anything. And, outside of the worry that comes with baby taking her first steps or the natural paranoia of losing a child in a shopping mall, many of the things we parents worry about are based on the natural parental instinct to protect our children. One of the resources many anxious parents often turn to for guidance is *Parents Magazine*. The publication is filled with tips about anything and everything related to parenting and over-parenting alike. One favorite topic the magazine covers is the percentile metrics that are often applied to chart the growth of a baby over time. One of the problems with these percentiles is that they don't account for ethnic differences. As noted in *Parents Magazine,* "babies of Asian, Hispanic, and Pacific Islander backgrounds tend to be smaller, on average, than babies of other ethnicities." The best advice, therefore, is to use percentiles only as a baseline. As Dr. Robert Eden, a clinical assistant professor of pediatrics at Brown University Medical School in Providence Rhode Island notes, "Your baby's position on the chart means very little to us . . . what matters is whether she's growing in a predictable trend." [151]

Learn More:

http://www.parents.com/baby/development/problems/baby-growing-normally/

AARP Works to Foster Technology Innovations for People 50+

A pioneer in the quest to inspire more innovation for those over 50, AARP has created an initiative to spark more collaboration among public and private groups working on technology solutions to solve the challenges people in this group care most about. One aspect of this initiative is a partnership with Startup Health, an organization that supports entrepreneurs and early-stage startup companies from around the world working in the health care industry. Projects like AARP's Innovation@50+ draw attention to and build more influential networks for those working to solve the problems of people of diverse age groups and populations using technology. Most importantly, AARP's effort may increase the visibility (and investment dollars) funneled toward health technologies, especially those suited for older adults.

Learn More:

http://www.aarp.org/technology/innovations/innovation-50-plus/about-innovation-50-plus/

http://medcitynews.com/2013/04/what-do-seniors-need-startup-health-and-aarp-collaboration-hopes-to-give-startups-better-insights/

---

[14] See Appendix I for more information about digihealth pulse.

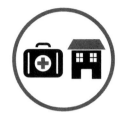

Trend 9:
Healthy Real Estate

Traditionally, people make choices about where they will live based on educational factors and a range of other amenities. In the future, more will use health and wellness criteria such as walkable communities, access to organic and local food sources, hospital ratings, and more to determine where they should buy or rent a home.

Ushi Okushima is perhaps the most famous centenarian in the world. Hailing from the Japanese prefecture of Okinawa, Okushima is just one of the hundreds of people from this area who are 100-plus years old. As populations around the world age, the task of learning how to keep people healthier and happier longer is becoming increasingly important. This is why researchers and others are studying Okushima and those like her to uncover their secrets.

One obvious place to start might be to interview Okushima to ask her what she believes is her secret to a long life. And when interviewers do that, Okushima credits her longevity to hard work, sleep and a nightly drink of mugwort sake; yet, asking centenarians to reveal their secrets may be a fool's game. Dan Buettner, author of the bestseller *The Blue Zones: Lessons for Living Longer From the People Who've Lived the Longest*, says centenarians "can no more tell us how they reached age 100 than a seven-foot man can tell us how he got to be so tall." [152]

So if we can't rely on centenarians to tell us why they age so well, how can we unlock their secrets? One way is to carefully study environmental, genetic, and societal characteristics common to those who live the longest. In his book, Buettner outlines nine tips for longer (and healthier) living based on traits shared by centenarians living around the world:

- **Move Naturally:** Engage in physical activity in ways that feel natural, rather than obligatory
- **Eat Less:** Cut unneeded calories by at least 20 percent
- **Favor Plants:** Eat less meat and processed food products
- **Drink Wine Daily:** One to two servings of wine is enough
- **Live With Purpose:** Be a big-picture thinker
- **Slow Down:** Reduce unhealthful stress in your life
- **Embrace Community:** Participate in spiritual activities with others
- **Family First:** Focus on being together with loved ones
- **Socialize With Others Who Share Similar Values:** Spend time with people who will reinforce rather than resist the life you choose to live

Looking at these nine tips, an interesting conclusion begins to emerge. While it may be tempting to look for a genetic explanation for long life, healthier living may have far more to do with communities and environments than genetics.

Individual Motivation is Not Enough: Why Livable Communities Are Vital to Health and Wellbeing

Buettner's advice may be nearly impossible for many readers to follow because of where they live. For example, sitting in traffic for hours commuting to and from work limits the amount of physical activity in which one can engage. Eating on the go, behind our desks, or at convenient, but unhealthful fast-food restaurants makes limiting calories difficult. And, living in areas with high crime, traffic, noise, or pollution can make Buettner's advice appear unrealistic, if not naïve.

For many years, those inside and outside of public health have recognized the important role communities play in fostering wellbeing. The government of the nation of Bhutan, for example, has long used a policy of measuring Gross National Happiness as the standard by which to make political and societal decisions for its citizens. The city of Toronto in Canada has turned to open data and government transparency in an effort to promote what it calls "neighborhood vibrancy." [153] And, in the United States, the government-backed initiative "Let's Move" has made it a priority to ensure that people living in cities and towns across the nation have access to healthful food and places to exercise.

The ability to engage in regular physical activity, such as walking to school and biking to work, is also heavily influenced by where one lives. This is a major reason why the walkable communities movement has gained traction in recent years. [154] According to the non-profit America Walks, pedestrian-friendly cities and towns are not only healthier, but have stronger economies and boast higher home prices. [155] In its 2009 study *Walking the Walk: How Walkability Raises Housing Values in U.S. Cities*, the group CEOs for Cities assigned ratings of 0 to 100 for factors such as proximity to amenities (i.e., restaurants, parks, schools, and stores) and concluded that a one-point increase in "Walk Score" corresponded to an increase of $700 to $3,000 in housing values, depending on the market. [156]

Traditionally, Americans have based decisions on where to purchase or rent homes on factors such the quality of the educational system and crime rates; however, recently, people have begun to place more importance on health-related factors, including access to parks, trails, and other facilities that enable them to improve their health and wellbeing.

According to a 2013 study produced by the National Association of Realtors, older adults tend to place greater emphasis on access to friends and family and health facilities when deciding where to purchase a home. [157] In addition, younger home purchasers (below age 33) were most likely to rate access to parks and other recreational activities as a major factor in their home buying decisions. [157]

A thirst for walkable communities will increasingly be drivers of where an aging American population chooses to live in the future. In a 2010 report, AARP documented this trend, noting that about half of respondents to its survey said "being somewhere where it's easy to walk [is] extremely or very important." [158]

The health and wellness industry is also measuring Americans' access to healthy real estate and working to make it a reality. For example, in 2008, Healthways (along with the polling organization Gallup) launched the Well-Being Index. One of the key aspects of the study is the Basic Access sub-index, which measures the availability of "necessities crucial to wellbeing" including "affordable fruits and vegetables," and a "safe place to exercise." [159]

In addition to the Well-Being Index, Healthways is producing a national initiative based on concepts outlined in Buettner's *Blue Zones Project*. Its goal is to foster the development of healthy communities by encouraging "permanent changes to environment, policy, and social networks" via the use of digital and analog technologies. [160] One major component of the project is the Blue Zones Certification initiative, a series of requirements that employers, restaurants, stores, and schools must meet to qualify as Blue Zone organizations. [161]

Apart from the research around walkable communities and the development of "Blue Zones" that we have shared in this chapter, healthy real estate also refers to changes in the design, development, and architecture of the buildings themselves. When you consider the innovations in green building and ergonomic structures that consider human wellbeing in their designs, you can see why architectural innovations are also influencing how people buy or rent real estate.

How Important is Healthy Real Estate to ePatients?

As outlined above, the healthy real estate trend is gaining steam. Given this, we wanted to see if health and wellness considerations were playing a role in ePatients' decisions about where to buy or rent a home and what this means for the future. To investigate, Enspektos asked ePatients participating in the 2013 edition of its digihealth pulse study:[15]

- Whether they had moved in the past two years, or were planning a move in the immediate future

- If they had moved/plan to move, whether the quality of nearby clinics or hospitals, the environment, access to food (such as organic/local), or other health and wellness factors played a minor, moderate, or major role in their decisions about where to live

Enspektos anticipated that health considerations would play some role in ePatients' moves, and we found this to be the case. Overall, a slight majority (52%) of ePatients (who had moved/were planning a move) said health and wellness factors played a role in where they decided to live (Figure XIV).

Enspektos was also interested in learning how the healthy real estate movement might take shape in the future. For example, are people in their mid-20s to 30s thinking about health issues when executing or planning a move?

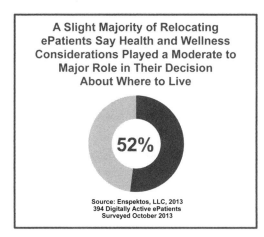

A Slight Majority of Relocating ePatients Say Health and Wellness Considerations Played a Moderate to Major Role in Their Decision About Where to Live

52%

Source: Enspektos, LLC, 2013
394 Digitally Active ePatients
Surveyed October 2013

Figure XIV: Percentage of ePatients Who Moved in the Past Two Years (or Planning a Move in the Near Future) Who Say Health and Wellness Factors Played a Moderate to Major Role in Their Decision About Where to Live

Overall, 30 percent of 25- to 34-year-olds and 23 percent of those aged 18 to 24 said health considerations played a moderate role in their moves. Among those saying health issues had a major impact, about one-third of this group were between 25 and 44 years old; however, this was a much smaller overall group—as only 13 percent of all relocating ePatients said health and wellness considerations had a major impact on their moves.

These results suggest that digital innovators, government officials, and real estate executives should be paying close attention to issues related to healthy real estate, as it is important today, but will become vital tomorrow, especially as people age.

Stories: Healthy Real Estate

Delos Dreams Up the WELL Building Standard

In terms of tapping the trend of people who want healthier homes to fit into their healthier communities, no real estate developer has been as forward thinking as Delos. The firm spearheaded the development of a now-globally accepted "Well Building Standard" that is designed to offer flexible guidelines for the addition of home building features that can positively impact health and wellness. Some of Delos' healthy real estate-related amenities include toxin filters, optimal lighting, and design and technology solutions for lowering stress, enabling healthier eating choices, and encouraging greater levels of physical activity. Sound ambitious? The developer has already built five "health-centric residences" at 66 East 11th Street in New York and founder Paul D. Scialla's personal loft has become a showcase, attracting tours from powerful patrons such as former President Bill Clinton and spiritual guru Deepak Chopra. Expanding the idea beyond just healthy homes, the MGM Grand hotel in Las Vegas also features first-ever "Stay Well Rooms" that add air purification, EMF protection, aromatherapy, and other luxury amenities for well-heeled guests.

Learn More:

http://delosliving.com/mission/well-building-standard/

http://www.nytimes.com/2013/06/30/realestate/health-centric-homes-for-a-price.html

http://www.mgmgrand.com/hotel/stay-well.aspx

Famed Technology Innovator Aims to Improve Community Health With Her HICCup Manifesto

In May 2013, former Wall Street analyst and noted technology futurist and investor, Esther Dyson published a manifesto designed to draw greater attention to one of the biggest challenges in health care: self-inflicted illnesses from bad eating habits and sedentary lifestyles. Simply telling people to change their habits doesn't work. Neither do fear-based messages—in the long term, at least. So what's the solution?

Dyson's manifesto advocates encouraging healthful behaviors by focusing on communities of fewer than 100,000 people. By facilitating change at a hyper-local level, policies can be enacted, grassroots groups can be supported, and collaboration can happen with limited bureaucracy—and ultimately unhealthful behaviors can be reduced. It is easy to overlook the real estate aspect of this master plan; yet, at its heart, the manifesto is inspired by the idea that also powers this trend: people thrive when they live in communities that truly support their health and wellbeing.

Learn More:

http://www.project-syndicate.org/commentary/how-communities-can-hold-down-health-care-costs-by-esther-dyson

http://www.technologyreview.com/news/518901/esther-dyson-we-need-to-fix-health-behavior/

Relocality: Using Social Data to Help People Relocate to Communities That Are Just Right—and Healthier

The real estate industry has seen plenty of disruption from technology, both in how people search for homes as well as in the process for deciding where to live. One of the most interesting of these new 2.0-style services is a startup called Relocality that uses the seldom-used, but poetically brilliant marketing tagline "Long to Belong No Longer" as a description for the services they offer. The tool connects to your social networking profiles and pulls thousands of features and preferences from your previous history, then uses this data to generate a list of "dimensions" for the criteria that might be important to you in deciding where to live. This data is crunched to identify the three most closely related neighborhoods that fit your parameters, which you may want to investigate further. While the idea is still new and hardly mainstream, the insight that a sense of "belonging" contributes to overall health and happiness is scientifically sound. And, the idea that emotional and spiritual wellness is directly related to physical wellness is one that sits at the heart of the healthy real estate trend.

Learn More: https://relocality.com/#how_does_relocality_do_it

---

[15] See Appendix I for more information about digihealth pulse.

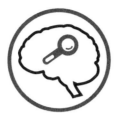

Trend 10:
Neuro-Influence Mapping

Advances in brain imaging technology offer new insights into patients' behavioral profiles to support the development of unique, personalized treatment programs that factor in which method of influence (fear, authority, conforming, etc.) may be most likely to work. Marketers are also using brain-mapping technologies for advertising purposes.

In 2013, the Institute of Education in London published a study that presented a bleak conclusion. According to data from standardized tests, the brightest children in England had results that ranked them two years behind their counterparts in Taiwan and Hong Kong by the time they reached the age of 16. [162]

A report from Harvard's Program on Education Policy and Governance (PEPG), a program designed to study the performance of U.S.-based students' performance in math similarly concluded that "the percentages of high-achieving math students in the U.S. —and most of its individual states—are shockingly below those of many of the world's leading industrialized nations." [163]

Blame for these dismal East vs. West performances in math typically fall on the usual culprits: teaching methods, lower academic standards, and lazy students.

But, what if the solution actually came down to something so simple many kids would probably describe it as a toy?

In a fascinating study published in the June 27, 2006 issue of *New Scientist*, researchers at Dalian University tested a combination of 12 local college seniors in the northeastern Chinese city of Dalian (native language Mandarin), as well as 12 English speakers from the United States, Australia, the United Kingdom, and Canada. Each volunteer was measured in a magnetic resonance imaging (MRI) machine as they solved math problems. [164]

The research showed similar activity in the parietal cortex (the region responsible for the sense of quantity) but as team member Eric Reiman from the Banner Good Samaritan Medical Center in Phoenix, Arizona, suggested, "Native English speakers [relied] more on additional brain regions involved in the meaning of words, whereas native Chinese speakers [relied] more on additional brain regions involved in the visual appearance and physical manipulation of numbers." [164]

Reiman and his colleagues theorized that the common practice in Asian schools of using an abacus might help students to think more visually about numbers, and the visual nature of the Mandarin language itself may impact native Chinese speakers' math ability as well. More importantly, as Barry Horwitz of the National Institute on Deafness and Other Communication Disorders (NIDCD) noted in the article, "The results do suggest that learning to read in a particular way—or more generally, the cultural differences associated with different language groups—may have an impact in other cognitive domains, in this case arithmetic processing." [164]

The debate about how much of our behavior is influenced by genetics versus the environment in which we grow is heated and never-ending; yet, the fascinating conclusion that the study above, as well as others looking at similar behaviors, are uncovering is that our environments may shape our personalities and our fundamental brain structures more than we realize.

Answering the question for sure, though, will take a far more sophisticated understanding of the brain than we currently have. Two major global initiatives currently underway are poised to accelerate the development of exactly this type of understanding of the brain. One is a European initiative known as the Human Brain Project. Funded as a 10-year, large-scale research initiative, its goal is to "understand the human brain and its diseases and ultimately to emulate its computational capabilities." [165] Another is the U.S.-based BRAIN (Brain Research Through Advancing Innovative Neurotechnologies) Initiative, described below.

The BRAIN Initiative

"As humans, we can identify galaxies light years away, we can study particles smaller than an atom. But, we still haven't unlocked the mystery of the three pounds of matter that sits between our ears." - President Barack Obama [166]

On April 2, 2013, President Barack Obama introduced a sweeping project, the BRAIN Initiative, designed to unlock the mysteries of the human brain. Comparing the BRAIN Initiative to the Human Genome Project, the president talked about how government investment in genetic research has resulted in significant benefits for many sectors of the economy and improved lives. [166]

The BRAIN Initiative comes on the heels of more than two decades of intensive interest, research, and reporting on neuroscience. Colorful scans of human brains regularly accompany news reports, articles, and books focusing on cognition, emotion, and more. The neuroscience boom was facilitated by two technologies: positron emission tomography (PET) and functional magnetic resonance imaging (fMRI). Both PET and fMRI enable scientists, technicians, and others to take snapshots or videos of brain activity and display them on computer screens. PET scans require the injection of a radioactive tracer into the brain. In contrast, fMRI is a non-invasive scanning technique that uses radio waves and magnets to measure blood flow to different parts of the brain in response to physical activity, pictures, and more.

"Imagine you had a device that allowed you to read people's minds," a 2007 publication on fMRI produced by the American Psychological Association begins. [167] This sentence captures the primary reason we have become so fascinated with fMRI technology. Because fMRI brain scans provide data suggesting that certain regions of the brain light up (or receive increased blood flow) in response to stimuli or activity, people have been using them to address long-unanswered questions about human behavior.

For example, psychologists and medical researchers have used fMRIs to:

- Determine what makes people happy, which can be used to fight depression using non-drug therapy [167]
- Reprogram the brains of people with conditions like dyslexia [167]
- Potentially identify conditions such as autism and attention deficit disorder (ADD) [168]
- Guide drug therapy for various mental illnesses such as schizophrenia and depression [168]

The volume of research being conducted with fMRI technology might lead some to question whether government investment in brain research is necessary. If we can use fMRI to measure and even predict behavior, why go deeper? Neuroscientists would answer this question by highlighting the limitations of fMRIs. Most importantly, although fMRI measures brain activity, it does not really tell us how the brain actually works.

Neuroscientist John Kubie has described this problem using computing terminology. "In order to understand how the brain functions (and subsequently why we do what we do), we need to unpack the brain's algorithms or programs that help us accomplish tasks like transforming images into meaning or coordinating activities taking place in different areas of the brain." [169] In other words, fMRI tells us what parts of the brain are being activated by the brain's programming, but nothing about the processes that drive it.

In an essay published in the *New Yorker* in 2012, Gary Marcus pointed out another limitation of fMRIs: their resolution. "The smallest element of a brain image that an fMRI can pick out is something called a voxel," he wrote. "But voxels are much larger than neurons, and, in the long run, the best way to understand the brain is probably not by asking which particular voxels are most active in a given process. It will instead come from asking how the many neurons work together within those voxels." [170]

Currently, the goals of the BRAIN Initiative are still taking shape. [171] Yet, it is clear that the project's focus will be to develop technologies and techniques that allow for a much deeper understanding of how individual neurons and various parts of the brain work together and separately to drive human behavior, cause or accelerate disease, and more. [172] Despite its limitations, fMRI will continue to be an important tool for understanding how the brain functions and predicting behavior.

Over the next few years, interest and analysis of brain function and behavior will accelerate as the BRAIN Initiative comes into greater focus and fMRI technology advances. In the following stories, we provide additional insights on how brain scanning technology will impact patient care, including in the area of mental illness, and how it is influencing marketing efforts.

Stories: Neuro-Influence Mapping

Neuro-Influence Meets NeuroMarketing

The most fundamental marketing question may be one you have heard many times before: Coke or Pepsi? It is the classic brand preference challenge; and soft drink makers have learned that people are notoriously bad at predicting which product they prefer. This is because most of us can't truly taste the difference between Coke and Pepsi as well as we think we can. In 2004, researchers at the Baylor College of Medicine gave 67 people the choice between the two brands and watched the resulting brain scans during the interaction. While more people preferred Pepsi in the blind taste test, when alerted about which was which, three out of every four chose Coke. The brain scans showed that when drinking Coke, not only were the reward parts of the brain craving the drink, but the memory regions also lit up. This is but one example of how neuromarketers have used brain scans to uncover the roots of human purchasing behavior.

Learn More:

http://content.time.com/time/magazine/article/0,9171,1580370,00.html

---

How Brain Mapping is Guiding Treatment for Mental Illnesses

One of the most powerful use cases for brain scanning is to understand better what influences people suffering from behavioral issues or mental illness. In one study, researchers worked to build an image of the brains of people with eating disorders to try and map the patterns that might lead to this problem. [173] Another study used brain mapping to understand alcohol's effects on first-year college students. [174] Yet another looked at the possibilities for how brain mapping and neurofeedback might help to treat attention deficit hyperactivity disorder in children. [175] What all of these studies illustrate is the dramatic potential for brain mapping to serve the same purposes that the Human Genome Project did in the world of genetics by offering practitioners a map from which to build their research efforts.

Using Buildings to Grow Our Brains and Inspire Innovation

At the 2003 American Institute of Architects Conference, neurobiologist Fred Gage presented some relatively surprising findings illustrating that our brains don't truly stop growing in our twenties, but instead that adults "grow" new neurons in response to their environment. [176] In his talk, he noted that "changes in the environment change the brain, and therefore they change our behavior." [176] It is a conclusion supported by a group called the Academy of Neuroscience for Architecture, which believes that some types of buildings and spaces can also result in the growth of new neurons, and therefore look at the important role that architecture can take in creating spaces that inspire great ideas and breakthroughs in culture and science.

Learn More:

http://www.psmag.com/culture/corridors-of-the-mind-49051/

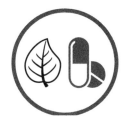

Trend 11:
Natural Medicine

Long called "alternative" medicine in a dismissive way by some health professionals, new science will continue to prove old beliefs about the value of spices, tonics, and herbs. The result will be more mainstream credibility for natural remedies that were once disbelievingly called "miracle cures," but now have a body of tangible results to prove their value once and for all.

Did alternative medicine kill Steve Jobs? This was the question of the moment after the Apple CEO and co-founder's untimely death from cancer. In his 2011 biography, Walter Isaacson revealed that after initially being told he had a neuroendocrine tumor in his pancreas, Jobs did not immediately undergo surgery, the accepted and recommended treatment for his condition. [177] Instead, Jobs told Isaacson that he had decided to "see if a few other things would work." Driven by a fear of having doctors open up his body and a lifelong interest in alternative health practices, Jobs:

> "[K]ept to a strict vegan diet with large quantities of fresh carrot and fruit juices . . . [H]e [also] added acupuncture, a variety of herbal remedies, and occasionally a few other treatments he found on the

Internet or by consulting people around the country, including a psychic." [177]

Against the advice of his family, friends, and doctors, Jobs tried a range of non-traditional treatments for nine months after his cancer diagnosis. It was only after a scan revealed his tumor had grown, that he finally decided to undergo surgery. Isaacson suggested Jobs came to regret his decision not to have the tumor removed earlier. [177]

For some, Jobs' flirtation with non-traditional therapies (and dubious treatments promoted via the Internet) was further evidence that complimentary and alternative medicines, or CAMs, are unproven, harmful and life-threatening. [178] Yet, despite widespread skepticism in the established medical community toward vitamin supplements, massage, acupuncture, herbs and other CAMs, these treatments are widely prescribed in many countries, including the United Kingdom. [179]

Celebrity aside, Jobs is far from the only person who has tried CAM for a range of illnesses, including cancer. Many people use these therapies in combination with standard treatments and vouch for their effectiveness. For example, a 2013 analysis published in the journal *PLOS One* indicates that "40% of the British public" believes homeopathic remedies and conventional medicines are equally effective. [179]

In the United States, the use of CAM is widespread. According to research conducted by the federal government, 38% of adults said they used alternative therapies during the previous 12 months in 2007. [180]

Older people are especially likely to use CAM. A survey fielded by AARP and the National Center for Complementary and Alternative Medicine (NCCAM) in 2011 revealed that "just over half (53%) of people 50 and older reported using CAM at some point in their lives, and nearly as many (47 percent) reported using it in the past 12 months." [181] Also, while the use of CAM is widespread, seniors tend to hide the fact they are using alternative therapies from physicians and other health care providers. [181]

Conducting and Communicating CAM Research: A Vital Need

So who is right about the effectiveness of these so-called alternative medicines?

The fact is, vitamins and other supplements (for example) have become vital parts of therapy, especially in the area of disease prevention. Over 30 years ago, a major clinical trial testing the benefits of folic acid supplementation was launched. The study was halted in 1991 after researchers had gathered conclusive evidence that folic acid helped prevent birth defects. [182]

Research on folic acid highlights how important it is to conduct rigorous studies to better understand whether and how CAM is effective. In addition, determining if herbal medications, vitamins, and other therapies are free of dangerous substances and whether they interact with prescription medicines is absolutely vital. Finally, communication is key. Medical professionals and the public cannot make informed decisions about CAM without relevant and trustworthy information.

Some segments of the medical establishment, policymakers, and others have long recognized the importance of conducting and communicating studies that increase understanding of the benefits and risks associated with CAMs. In fact, a 2005 report published by the National Academy of Sciences outlined how the volume of CAM studies steadily increased between 1982 and 2002. [183]

This increase in CAM research is part of the reason we believe the natural medicine trend will accelerate over the next few years. Other reasons for this include:

- **Alternative Therapies May Help Reduce Medical Spending:** For many health systems, both in the United States and globally, reducing medical spending is a priority. One way to achieve this goal is by keeping people — especially if they have serious conditions — out of the hospital. Can vitamins and other therapies help? A 2013 analysis supported by a supplement industry trade group suggests that asking people with certain conditions such as heart disease to take vitamins may reduce health costs. [184] While this finding needs to be backed up by independent studies, it may spark additional research on the cost-savings benefits of vitamins and efforts to increase their use.

• **Government Agencies Are Committed to Supporting CAM Research and Communicating Balanced Data**: Established in 1998, the National Center for Complementary and Alternative Medicine (NCCAM), conducts research and delivers education on alternative therapies. In its third strategic plan, NCCAM outlined how it plans to use a range of communications channels to distribute "objective, evidence-based information on CAM interventions." Another NCCAM objective is to help health providers and others better understand how CAM is being used in the real world. The agency also wants to guide more productive conversations between patients and physicians on CAM use. [185] These activities may boost acceptance of CAM in established medical circles and make people more comfortable communicating about alternative therapies with health providers.

• **CAM Use May Increase As the Population Ages**: As discussed previously, older people are more likely to use CAM treatments. Use of these therapies will likely accelerate as the population ages, which will continue to boost the CAM industry and physicians' needs to understand these therapies.

• **Digital Tools Will Increase Knowledge**: As in other areas of health, digital technologies such as mobile and social media will likely increase the public's knowledge of CAM, especially when information is shared after first being communicated via mainstream media sources. Digital content about CAM may also shift how people use certain treatments as evidence emerges about their benefits and harms. For example, between 2000 and 2001, use of St. John's Wort decreased significantly after media reports and studies indicated it might make certain prescription medications less effective. [183]

Overall, there is still much to be done to help the medical establishment and patients increase their understanding of the benefits, harms, and uses of alternative therapies; however, as additional credible evidence emerges supporting CAM, patients and providers will become more skilled at separating fact from fiction.

Another factor impacting how people view "natural" foods and remedies is the global fascination with our distant past. Breads and granola are sold with "ancient" grains. Food labels scream that they are "All-Natural" and the idea that "organic" or anything more connected to nature must be better for you is becoming widespread.

This global embrace of the power of nature is also seeping into attitudes toward medical treatment as well. Some women insist on a natural childbirth despite the easy availability of pain-killing drugs. For many years, "Dead Sea Therapy" where patients lie in the sun and float in the Dead Sea in Israel has been shown to provide relief—after prolonged exposure—to sufferers of psoriasis in a way that most medicines have been unable to match. [186]

Diets, too, have seen the impact of this attitudinal return to the benefits of nature—as recent popular Western diets and weight loss trends have included the "Paleo Diet," the "Mediterranean Diet," the "Raw Food Diet" and many others. Some may work and others may not; yet, the prevailing belief is that the closer these treatments, diets, and products can come to truly being inspired by and derived from nature, the better.

The final aspect of the natural medicine movement that we would like to discuss—and explore through research—is the impact of the Web on ePatients' opinions about the value of natural therapies.

Has the Web Changed ePatients' Opinions of Natural Remedies?

As established by research from the Pew Research Center and other groups, the Internet can have a significant influence on how people perceive health and wellness issues; however, there is little information about how the Web is affecting what people think about natural remedies. Investigating this issue is important, as the changing opinions (either negative or positive) about CAM therapies may influence whether people decide to use these treatments and, hence, impact the popularity of the natural medicine movement.

Enspektos took a look at this question in the 2013 edition of its digihealth pulse study.[16] The firm asked ePatients whether information they had seen on the Web (over the past two years) about natural therapies made their opinions about these remedies worse, better, or if it had no impact on their thinking. (ePatients could also select "I Don't Know.")

Many ePatients (43%) said Web content improved their opinions of natural medicines (Figure XV). Only 8% reported that Internet information made it worse.

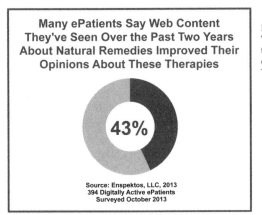

Many ePatients Say Web Content They've Seen Over the Past Two Years About Natural Remedies Improved Their Opinions About These Therapies

43%

Source: Enspektos, LLC, 2013
394 Digitally Active ePatients
Surveyed October 2013

Figure XV: Percentage of ePatients Who Say Information They've Seen on the Web About Natural Health Remedies Improved Their Opinions of These Therapies

Should public health experts, health providers, and others be worried about these results? Perhaps. As indicated by Steve Jobs' experience, many of the natural therapies that rank high in Web search results may be ineffective or unsafe; however, these survey results also represent an opportunity. Government organizations like the National Center for Complementary and Alternative Medicine have made it a priority to use the Web and other digital channels to communicate unbiased, research-based information to the public. By using the Web in smart ways, this federal agency and other groups are beginning to shape people's thinking about natural remedies using credible data.

This research also suggests that the natural medicine movement is gaining ground. In an interview about the dramatic growth in popularity of more holistic treatments, Benjamin Kligler, M.D. of the Continuum Center for Health and Healing at Beth Israel Medical Center in New York noted that his institution "sees roughly 4,000 patients per year and we can't see all the patients that want to come in." What is the major barrier holding back the tide of this demand for natural and alternative remedies? According to Kligler, "concerns over 'standard[s] of practice' are a major source of inhibition. We are prisoners of 'standards of care.'" [187]

In discussing the current situation, Kligler used the example of NSAIDs, such as aspirin, which have the known side effect of stomach bleeding, but are prescribed regardless; however, if doctors recommend herbs, and it causes an adverse event, he wondered whether this decision would be "supported by standards of care." He also notes there are "not a lot of cases of doctors getting sued for discussing or recommending herbs. In fact, [doctors] might encounter liability by not talking about them." [187]

It should be noted that inhibitions regarding herbs and other alternative treatments is a problem unique to Western medicine. Patients in Asian countries, for example, are far more likely to demand natural medical treatments and doctors are very willing to prescribe them.

Ultimately, globalization itself may be the driving force that leads more natural medicines toward becoming mainstream, and provides perhaps the greatest evidence to support the trend outlined in this chapter. Just as using feng shui for building design or turning to yoga as the preferred form of exercise were once foreign concepts, natural medicine too is experiencing a surge in popularity and belief from people ready and willing to use them.

Stories: Natural Medicine

Turmeric: A Wonder Spice Takes the World by Storm

For years, one of us (Rohit) grew up with turmeric as a key ingredient in everything from Indian curries to yogurt (partly as a cure for indigestion). In the past decade, people living outside of India have slowly discovered turmeric. Now routinely listed among the "world's healthiest foods," turmeric has significant anti-inflammatory properties that have been shown through some studies to be comparable to hydrocortisone creams and over-the-counter drugs such as Motrin. [188] Other studies have even cited turmeric as a possible reason for the lower rates of childhood leukemia observed in Asian versus Western countries. [189] Sales of turmeric have accelerated as understanding of the spice's medicinal benefits has increased. In 2012, data from the SPINSscan Report showed that, in the single herb category, "turmeric/curcumin products took six of the top 10 best-selling spots." [190] As the herb becomes more popular, prices continue to rise. Turmeric has also become one of the fastest growing exports from India to the rest of the world.

The Daniel Plan: Using Christianity to Fight Obesity

According to data from the Centers for Disease Control (CDC), somewhere between 29.8 and 42.7 percent of people age 20 or older living in a handful of states in the Southeastern and South-central United States are obese. [191] This region of America is often also called the "Bible Belt" because "socially conservative evangelical Protestantism is a significant part of the culture and Christian church attendance across the denominations is generally higher than the nation's average." [192] This overlap inspired a faith-based solution to the problem from an unlikely group of people. Noted functional medicine specialist and best selling author Dr. Mark Hyman, brain health expert Dr. Daniel Amen, and heart surgeon/television doctor Mehmet Oz, M.D. teamed up to develop a lifestyle plan based on the story of Daniel, who, according to the Bible "forsook the king's rich food in order to honor God's best for him and his friends." [193]

While the blame for poor eating habits can hardly be linked to religion, it may be faith that helps people adopt a healthier lifestyle. The Daniel Plan recommends people adopt more healthful eating habits and embrace treatments and diets based on nature. More importantly, it has been embraced by hundreds of churches and faith-based groups across the Bible Belt, and has the potential to affect more lasting change for people suffering from chronic illness and obesity in the region than almost any other diet. And so, for that reason, we chose to include it here as a powerful story of how natural medicine can help accelerate lifestyle and community change based on something as powerful and inspiring as religious faith.

Learn More: http://www.danielplan.com/whatistheplan

Plant-Based Sweetener Stevia Becomes a Sensation

The popular plant-based sweetener stevia has been dramatically growing in sales since being approved by the U.S. Food and Drug Administration in 2008. In fact, stevia's sales may reach between $1 and $2 billion in 2014. Stevia-based Truvia is currently the number-two brand of sugar substitute in the world, having already overtaken Equal and Sweet 'N Low. And, the product has even made appearances in pop culture. For example, it became a key element in the plot of the hit U.S. drama Breaking Bad.

Learn More:

http://www.nutraceuticalsworld.com/issues/2012-07/view_features/2012-international-herb-botanical-trends/

http://www.nutraceuticalsworld.com/issues/2013-10/view_industry-news/herbal-supplement-sales-grow-to-56-billion/

---

[16] See Appendix I for more information about digihealth pulse.

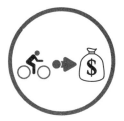

Trend 12:
MicroHealth Rewards

Inspired by U.S. federal legislation and a deeper understanding of behavioral science, insurers, corporations, health providers, and others will apply game theory to encourage people to adopt and sustain healthy behaviors by offering them tangible rewards (or punishments) as incentives.

Whether they are conscious of it or not, many parents spend a lot of time thinking about human behavior—and how to shape it. They quickly learn that creating rituals, providing detailed instructions, and offering rewards (and punishments) are the keys to controlling their children's impulses and (hopefully) turning them into well-behaved, socially acceptable adults.

In fact, some parents (and teachers) turn to star charts, which Alain de Botton describes in his book *Religion for Atheists: A Non-believer's Guide to the Uses of Religion*, as "complex domestic political settlements (usually to be found fastened to the sides of fridges or the doors of larders) which set forth in exhaustive detail the specific behaviours [sic] they expect from, and will reward in, their children." [194]

Star charts are an example of a behavior-modification approach that incentivizes positive actions using rewards. Star charts feature lists of desired behaviors (or rules) parents would like their children to follow. When children obey these rules, they receive a star and are often encouraged to collect a certain number in order to receive a reward. For example, if little Ravi cleans his room for a week, he will earn a gold star per day. If he earns five stars between Monday and Friday, he will be allowed to play video games on Saturday night.

Parents using star charts quickly learn they are highly effective. This is because children who receive instant visual feedback on their behavior are more likely to follow the rules. Star charts can also be used to shape behavior by encouraging healthy competition, as siblings will sometimes compete with each other to earn more stars and rewards.

In his book *Religion for Atheists*, de Botton wonders if adults might benefit from star charts. [194] He asked whether people would be less apt to behave badly if they knew their actions were being monitored and could earn rewards for good behavior. It turns out this idea may be more powerful than any of us realize.

Increasingly, employers, governments, and others are producing (and encouraging the development of) initiatives where people are provided with detailed instructions and rewards/punishments to incentivize them to act in certain ways in the areas of health and wellness. We refer to this trend as MicroHealth Rewards.

Those developing MicroHealth Rewards initiatives:

- Recognize that health, at its core, is defined by the rituals, or habits we follow on a daily basis, e.g., such as whether Ahmed consistently eats fruits and vegetables or potato chips. They also understand that asking people to exchange negative (and enjoyable) health rituals for positive ones is very difficult.
- Apply concepts from game theory to motivate people to action. Some forms of game theory operate under the assumption that most people are fundamentally rational beings who make decisions after analyzing the cost/benefits of their actions. Given this, providing people with opportunities to compete

or cooperate with others may shape short- and long-term health behaviors.

The Three Pillars of the MicroHealth Rewards Movement: Games, Technology, and Legislation

The MicroHealth Rewards movement is being driven by the convergence of three inter-related trends:

1. **The Gamification of Health:** Techniques developed by game makers are being applied to health in a quest to educate and change behavior
2. **Always-On Health Monitoring:** Tools or sensors that constantly track health activities (diet, exercise, etc.) can be used to monitor how people are managing their health
3. **The Use of Legislation to Motivate Health Behavior Change:** In the United States, the Affordable Care Act (or Obamacare) allows corporations, insurers, and others to provide people with rewards (and punishments) for engaging in certain health behaviors or participating in corporate wellness initiatives

These trends are described further below.

The Gamification of Health

World of Warcraft (WoW) is the most successful massively multiplayer online (MMO) game in history. Launched nearly a decade ago, WoW boasted nearly 12 million subscribers at its peak in 2010. Although its popularity is waning (as of May 2013, the number of WoW subscribers had fallen to 8 million) it is still very popular, especially in Asia. [195] This fantasy game enables players to take on a range of identities (from wizards to warriors), fight powerful enemies, and embark on epic quests to earn fame and fortune.

Blizzard, the company behind WoW, keeps subscribers paying month after month using a skillfully produced combination of:

- **Rewards:** Players spend a lot of time killing monsters and completing quests in order to level up their characters and earn more powerful skills, items, and abilities. This work-reward cycle is what keeps people playing the game, even during periods when it isn't very much fun.
- **Community:** Games like WoW are rarely played alone. Many players join guilds or groups of players who work together to earn items, complete quests, and more. Gamers form strong bonds with others playing the game, which keeps them engaged and active.
- **Punishments:** One drawback to the community aspect of WoW is that players who do not steadily progress in the game risk being left behind as their fellow gamers complete quests and earn items they cannot.

By the early 2000s, around the time that massive multiplayer online properties like WoW were emerging, the video game industry was changing and becoming increasingly profitable—and popular. With millions of people playing games online, using mobile devices and more, some began to look at whether techniques employed by developers of games like WoW could be used to educate and change health behavior.

One of the people examining this issue was Ben Sawyer, the co-founder of the game consultancy Digitalmill. In 2004, Sawyer, with the support of the Robert Wood Johnson Foundation, launched the Games for Health Project, an outgrowth of the Serious Games Initiative. [196]

Games for Health (primarily via its annual conference) has helped to centralize and spread the knowledge of designers, health organizations, and others using games to encourage healthy behaviors. Another consequence of Sawyer's efforts is that the popularity of incorporating rewards, community, and entertainment into health-focused games, wellness initiatives, software, and devices has steadily increased over the past few years. Today, when people talk about using gaming techniques (rewards, community, and punishments) to spark health behavior change—especially outside the realm of games—they often use the phrase "the gamification of health."

Health insurance firms have been quick to adopt gamification, employing it to boost engagement with mobile-fitness applications and more. For example, in 2010, UnitedHealthcare launched OptumizeMe, a mobile app designed to help people achieve various nutritional and fitness goals via the use of virtual badges "as rewards for participation and encouragement" and a social network where people can collaborate or compete with others. [197]

Using Sensors and Tracking Devices to Aid Health Gamification

The flip side is that inspiring people to adopt healthier behaviors through the power of gaming may not be as easy as we hoped. One significant barrier to health gamification is that it can take a lot of effort for people to manually track their activities, especially those related to diet and exercise. Luckily, over the past few years, a range of technologies has emerged that are not only making self-tracking easier, but are aiding the widespread implementation of health gamification efforts. Some of these include:

- **GPS:** One way to measure whether people are frequenting the gym, walking, etc. is to use a tracking technology available on most smartphones (and a growing number of fitness devices): GPS. For example, the Nike+ Sport-Watch GPS tracks users' locations, distances, and more. This information can be used to monitor progress against fitness goals and integrated into an overall wellness initiative.
- **Wearable Sensors:** Devices that track health status indicators, such as heart rate, sleep patterns, steps walked, and more are called sensors, which are being integrated into a range of popular devices, such as the Fitbit. Some companies are starting to use sensing devices (along with gamification) to encourage employees to improve their health. For example, in 2013, Tasting Table, which produces a daily food e-mail service, asked employees to voluntarily use the Jawbone UP sensor and compete in health challenges. The CEO of the company held a contest where the first person to walk more than 10,000 steps would receive free fitness classes. [198]

It is possible that, as technology advances, wearable-sensing devices such as smart watches and eyewear (like Google Glass) could also be used to accelerate health gamification via more intensive monitoring. For example, Chris Hol-lindale, founder of the startup Zesty has speculated that one day "Google Glass [could be used to] record all the food you ate, the portion sizes, and how much food you left on your plate. Suddenly, you'd have cracked the food-tracking problem and you'd have a massive opportunity to gamify and fix our increasing battle with preventable, diet-related health problems."[17] [199]

How Legislation is Being Used to Incentivize Healthy Behaviors

As powerful as its potential is, gamification is only one of the ways rewards and punishments are being used to encourage healthy behaviors. Another method is to raise or decrease health-insurance premiums depending on whether people exercise, quit smoking, and more.

In the United States, the Affordable Care Act is driving the rise of MicroHealth Rewards initiatives tied to health insurance or wellness programs. Two of the most important are:

1. **Charging Smokers Higher Premiums:** According to a 2013 Gallup poll, 58% of Americans said they backed the concept of insurance companies charging smokers higher rates. [200] Given the high level of support for penalizing smokers financially, it is perhaps no surprise that the Affordable Care Act allows health insurers to charge smokers up to 50% more on their premiums. This is because tobacco users use more health and medical services due to cancer and other smoking-related conditions. The hope is that financial penalties will motivate people to quit. [201]
2. **Offering Health Insurance Rebates to Those Participating in Wellness Programs:** Although workplace wellness programs are popular, it can be difficult to get employees to participate in these initiatives. (There are also questions about whether they actually reduce medical spending.) Partly in an effort to boost workers' engagement in wellness programs, the Affordable Care Act allows businesses to reward those participating in certain initiatives with a discount of 30% off their insurance-premium costs, which works out to about $1,600 per year, per worker. [202]

Offering Rewards for Healthy Behavior: Incredibly Valuable or Fundamentally Flawed?

The practice of using rewards and punishments to encourage healthy behaviors has much support within the health community and will accelerate over the coming years; however, some question exists as to whether it is wholly ethical to incorporate gamification into health or penalize people financially for their behaviors.

One of the leaders of this contrarian view is Bonnie Henry, who heads the gaming company, GameMetrix Solutions. She warns that simply giving people points or rewards for participation "is not sustaining." She argues that "the deep elements of games [is] what makes them motivating." [203] Michael Fergusson, CEO of Canada-based health-games firm Ayogo, has a similar opinion. At the 2012 mHealth Summit he said: "Bribery is not a game. It's not enough just to give people rewards for doing the right thing." [204]

Others question whether it is ethical to charge higher health premiums to those who smoke or are overweight. They suggest this practice may discourage those who need health insurance the most—such as the poor—from seeking coverage. For example, writing in *Bioethics Forum*, David Resnick, a bioethicist at the National Institute for Environmental Health Sciences, said: "Since smokers tend to have significantly lower incomes than non-smokers, they could be especially vulnerable to increased health-insurance costs. If smokers opt out of health insurance this could have a detrimental impact on their access to health care and negatively impact their health . . . It would be ironic—and tragic—if charging smokers higher health insurance rates prevented them from accessing services that could help them stop smoking." [205]

At the end of the day, the most effective way to use financial incentives in health may be to recognize that they do work, but only over the short term. Because of this, rewards should be used in combination with other behavior-change strategies. In an interview conducted for this book, Nedra Weinreich, a health-behavior change expert and author of *Hands-On Social Marketing: A Step-by-Step Guide to Designing Change for Good*, told us:

"Incentives—especially financial ones—can be very persuasive for behavior change. When attuned to what the participants want, they can motivate someone to adopt healthy behaviors like starting a new exercise program or stopping smoking.

In the short term, as long as the incentives keep flowing, the change is likely to stick; however, research has shown that in many cases, once the initial incentive is gone, long-term change for its own sake is less likely to continue. Much more effective than that, extrinsic motivation is cultivating internal reasons to make the change and keep it going. This might include tying the behavior to an individual's core values and giving them the autonomy to determine the method that works best for them. Creating the conditions that allow people to motivate themselves will help to build sustainable behavior change— through making the behavior socially desirable, finding ways to make the behavior as easy as possible, and changing the environment."

ePatients and MicroHealth Rewards Initiatives

As outlined above, we know that MicroHealth Rewards programs have been growing in popularity over the past few years, but how many ePatients are currently in them and who might be targets for these initiatives in the future? To find out, Enspektos asked ePatients participating in the 2013 edition of its digihealth pulse study the following question: "Have you ever been offered a reward such as money, discounts, or something else in exchange for losing weight, quitting smoking, or taking another action related to your health?"[18]

Overall, Enspektos found that a minority of ePatients (12%) report having been offered rewards in exchange for engaging in healthy behaviors (Figure XVI); however, in a trend with significant implications for the future, those with chronic conditions such as high blood pressure and diabetes were more likely to report participating in MicroHealth Rewards initiatives (Figure XVII). This certainly makes sense, as offering rewards to less healthy people in exchange for losing weight, or controlling their diabetes using diet and exercise might yield the most benefits.

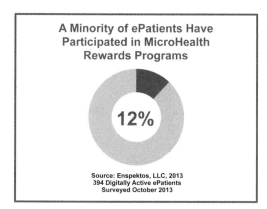

A Minority of ePatients Have Participated in MicroHealth Rewards Programs

12%

Source: Enspektos, LLC, 2013
394 Digitally Active ePatients
Surveyed October 2013

Figure XVI: Percentage of ePatients Who Have Participated in Programs Rewarding Them for Engaging in Healthy Behavior

Figure XVII: Percentage of ePatients Who Have Participated in Programs Rewarding Them for Engaging in Healthy Behavior (by Chronic Condition Status)

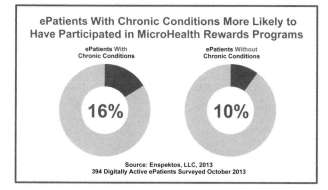

ePatients With Chronic Conditions More Likely to Have Participated in MicroHealth Rewards Programs

ePatients With Chronic Conditions

16%

ePatients Without Chronic Conditions

10%

Source: Enspektos, LLC, 2013
394 Digitally Active ePatients Surveyed October 2013

Stories: MicroHealth Rewards

Will Kinect Expand the Boundaries of Health Technology Innovation?

Marcelo Calbucci is the Co-Founder and CTO of EveryMove, a startup in Seattle working with health plans, gyms, brands, and employers by rewarding individuals for their healthy lifestyles. He is also a former development manager at Microsoft and one of the most enthusiastic believers in the potential power of the Kinect, which works with the Xbox One gaming system and provides motion-tracking and controller-free gaming. In an article published in May of 2013, Calbucci said "no other device, with the exception of the smartphone, will do more for the evolution of health technology than the Kinect 2.0 on the new Xbox One." [206] Why is he so excited? Thanks to new innovative features that allow for heart-rate monitoring, integration with high-resolution digital cameras, high-fidelity microphones, and (most importantly) a well-conceived software platform for game developers to build into . . . the Kinect 2.0 on the Xbox One and future devices will allow for new possibilities in the world of virtual fitness and fitness gaming. As these devices wirelessly connect to the Internet, there will be hundreds of opportunities for integration, live tracking, and rewards that health care institutions or employers can offer based on the principles of gamification.

Learn More: https://everymove.org/

StickK: Fail to Meet a Public Commitment and Pay—Happily

Yale University Professor Dean Karlan had an epiphany several years ago about how and why people might achieve their most difficult personal goals by making public commitments. Inspired, he thought of developing a Web site called StickK that allows anyone to use this behavioral technique to make public commitments funded by real dollars that are paid or donated the moment they fail to follow through.

Teaming up with then Yale student Jordan Goldberg, StickK was born. Over the past several years, multiple media have covered how StickK uses a powerful methodology to help people achieve all sorts of goals. Some meet their objectives through competition with friends. Others motivate themselves by triggering automatic donations to causes or politicians they hate every time they fail to achieve a milestone. At its heart, StickK is built on simple gamification principles and the idea that the promise of incentives (even if they happen to be negative) can be powerful motivators to commit to and stick with behavior change.

Learn More: http://www.stickk.com/about.php

---

[17] For a discussion of the drawbacks of self-tracking and health-quantification technologies, please see trend #6: The Over-Quantified Self.

[18] See Appendix I for more information about digihealth pulse.

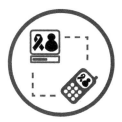

Part 3:
Digital Peer-to-Peer Health Care:
Harnessing the Social Web for Support, Knowledge, and Research

"I've said it before and I'll say it again: the most exciting innovation of the connected health era is . . . people talking with each other."

— Susannah Fox, Pew Research Center [42]

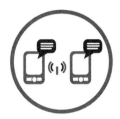

Trend 13:
Virtual Counseling

People are using online tools to seek and forge one-on-one relationships and offer virtual logistical and emotional support. This can include helping others to navigate the new health-insurance landscape, "sponsoring," or counseling one another and providing unique knowledge about conditions, ailments, and caregiving.

In 2004, Katherine Stone launched her blog, *Postpartum Progress*, with these words: "There are still women who can't get treatment because they either don't have insurance or what they have covers little to no psychiatric care. There are still women killing themselves and/or others. There are still women being undiagnosed or misdiagnosed. This can't continue to go on. I hope [this blog] helps in some small way." [207]

Little did Stone know that her modest blog would become a safe haven and a lifeline for mothers around the world experiencing postpartum depression. Stone's site is much more than an information source, it has saved lives. "I was in so much pain and was detached from who I really was," one reader wrote to Stone. "I read your article about hospitalization and I knew that was what I needed. I held you in my mind and was honest with my doctor. She recommended in-patient treatment . . . You have given me the strength to pull all of my pride to the side and step out to become a stronger mom." [208]

Stone decided to write *Postpartum Progress* after experiencing postpartum depression and learning how few resources were available for mothers with this condition. Stone is a prime example of how patients, caregivers, and others have become *de facto* counselors who play an important role in how people are educated about and manage their health and wellbeing. In this chapter, we focus on the rise in quantity and influence of these individuals through a trend we call *Virtual Counseling*.

Despite our belief in the importance of virtual counseling, the majority of conversations about how people use the Web for health have primarily focused on its role as an information source. Clearly, health information seeking is a far more common health-related task for people to engage in online than joining communities to find like-minded individuals or fellow patients suffering from the same illnesses; yet, the Web is increasingly becoming more than a popular source for information on treatments and advice.

We see that today a number of factors are already combining to raise the Web's profile as a virtual counseling resource (specifically, either giving or receiving emotional/moral support). Here are a few reasons why this is happening:

- Changes in the Health-Insurance Landscape: As health care legislation continues to evolve in multiple countries, ordinary people are teaching themselves to navigate the system and sharing their personalized expertise with others. The silver lining in this increasingly complex world of insurance coverage is that helpful people have turned to the Web and social media to provide information and support to others.

- Increase in the Chronic Disease and Caregiver Populations: The Pew Research Center and other organizations have reported that those with chronic conditions and caregivers are more likely to use the Web and social media to seek support. As the population grows and ages, the number of caregivers and people with long-term conditions will increase. These demographic changes are likely to boost the rate of (and necessity for) virtual counseling in the future.

ePatients and Virtual Counseling

Although the Pew Research Center has looked at the question of whether people go online to find information and support from others, there is still more to be learned about this topic. Specifically, are ePatients using the Web to provide emotional or moral assistance to others—or seeking it for themselves?

To answer this question, Enspektos asked ePatients participating in the 2013 edition of its digihealth pulse study whether they had ever engaged in virtual-counseling activities.[19]

This was defined as either:

- Receiving emotional or moral support via the Web or social sites from someone else
- Offering assistance (emotional or moral) to another person via the Internet or social media

Perhaps unsurprisingly—given that Enspektos surveyed ePatients—the majority (56%) said they had engaged in virtual counseling related activities (Figure XVIII). This statistic suggests that providing, as well as seeking, emotional and moral support online is a common activity for ePatients.

Figure XVIII: Percentage of ePatients Who Have Provided/Received
Emotional or Moral Support via the Web and Social Media

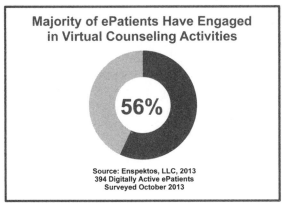

**Majority of ePatients Have Engaged
in Virtual Counseling Activities**

56%

Source: Enspektos, LLC, 2013
394 Digitally Active ePatients
Surveyed October 2013

Currently, people are offering (and seeking) support to those using the
health-insurance exchanges mandated by the U.S. Affordable Care Act. [209]
We were curious to see if ePatients who had previously used or were planning
on using the exchanges were more likely to have participated in virtual counseling activities.

In the 2013 edition of digihealth pulse, Enspektos asked ePatients if they had
already used or were planning on using the exchanges in the future. After controlling for planned/previous participation, Enspektos found that those interested in the exchanges were about 10% more likely to report participating in
virtual counseling activities (Figure XIX).[20]

This data suggests that ePatients using the exchanges may be much more open
to seeking or providing peer support (via the Web and social media).

Figure XIX: Percentage of ePatients Who Have Provided/Received
Emotional or Moral Support via the Web and Social Media
(by Previous or Planned Health-Insurance Exchange Participation Status)

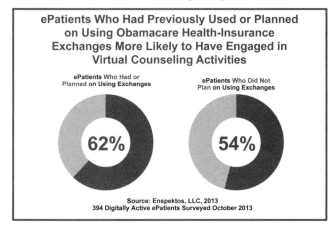

ePatients Who Had Previously Used or Planned on Using Obamacare Health-Insurance Exchanges More Likely to Have Engaged in Virtual Counseling Activities

ePatients Who Had or Planned on Using Exchanges

ePatients Who Did Not Plan on Using Exchanges

62%

54%

Source: Enspektos, LLC, 2013
394 Digitally Active ePatients Surveyed October 2013

Stories: Virtual Counseling

Caring.com: Supporting the Caregivers of Alzheimer's Patients and More

The global rise in Alzheimer's-related dementia is projected to reach 277 million by 2050 and will affect more than those individuals forced to battle this degenerative disease. [210] Alzheimer's may also contribute to a global shortage in caregivers, the families, loved ones, and professionals who are responsible for providing care outside a medical facility to patients as they age.

Caring.com is one of several online communities designed specifically to help caregivers provide support via a range of resources, including tips and advice for managing medications and tools that facilitate the search for care providers. The market opportunity in this space, with more than 50 million people in the United States alone playing the role of caregivers, is vast and Caring.com is one of the most comprehensive tools available for people assuming the important role of caregiver.

Learn More: http://www.caring.com

Smart Patients: Leveraging Health Care's Most Underutilized Resource

The Smart Patients project is motivated by a single, powerful belief: patients are the most underutilized resource in health care. Founded by online health community pioneer Gilles Frydman and former Google Chief Health Strategist Roni Zeiger, M.D., Smart Patients aims to "tap into the knowledge created by networks of engaged patients" to bring together collective conversations among cancer patients and caregivers alike about the effectiveness of treatments and ongoing clinical trials.

In addition, from a virtual counseling perspective, users can seek and provide support and knowledge. What makes the community especially powerful is that topics such as how treatments are performing are not off limits; moreover, Smart Patients' clinical trial search engine and database is a powerful tool people are using to find studies and share information about medical research with others.

Learn More: https://www.smartpatients.com/

Crohnology: Filling the Vast Information and Support Gap for People With Crohn's and Colitis

Sean Ahrens was diagnosed with Crohn's disease at the young age of 12. Seeking information on the disease at the time he realized there was little knowledge available about his rare condition and online support for people with it. This educational and virtual counseling gap motivated Sean to co-found Crohnology.

Sean has the ambitious goal of collecting the experiences of Crohn's patients and building a patient-powered research network that will allow them to guide research. As of this writing, Crohnology is currently available to people with Crohn's or colitis, seeking education, emotional support, and more.

Learn More: https://crohnology.com/

---

[19] See Appendix I for more information about digihealth pulse.
[20] Enspektos launched the 2013 edition of digihealth pulse on October 17, 2013. The health exchanges became active on October 1.

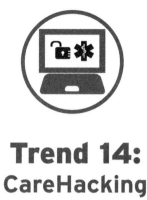

Trend 14:
CareHacking

As patient health data becomes more widely available and the number of caregivers managing medical care for family members increases, digitally savvy health consumers will leverage the information they gain from doctors, the Web, and other sources to better "hack" the health system to educate themselves, navigate loopholes, find more efficiencies, and ultimately get better, lower-cost and faster care for themselves and those they love.

Xeni Jardin, reeling from a recent breast cancer diagnosis, had finally accessed the files containing medical scans of her bones and other parts of her body. The images she found were both fascinating and shocking—especially when she saw a "ghost-like" penis superimposed on her leg. [211]

Jardin, editor, writer, and producer at the popular Web site *Boing Boing*, soon learned that she had not grown a male reproductive organ because she had been given someone else's health data files. But, her CareHacking experience also taught Jardin an important lesson: health is information rich, but data quality is sometimes poor.

In this chapter, we use Jardin's experiences and data collected from ePatients to describe three aspects of the CareHacking trend:

1. **Improving Patient Access to Medical Data:** Global trends in digitizing health information and legislation is helping many health-care providers move from paper-based to digital records and improving patients' ability to access their data in digital format.
2. **Guiding Care Using Personal Data:** Having access to data is not enough; patients need to use it to guide and improve their care.
3. **Using Knowledge Gained via the Web to Better Navigate the Health System:** We know ePatients (and caregivers) are using the Web to find health information, but is the knowledge they're gaining helping them find affordable health care, get treatment faster, and more? Yes.

More People Are Accessing Their Data, But We Still Have a Long Way to Go

Jardin's story is instructive because patients, caregivers, and others are going to receive more exposure to their personal medical data. As health data becomes more accessible to health consumers, the CareHacking trend will accelerate because this information will help people better understand what's happening inside their bodies and how to better manage their care; however, there is also a drawback to greater health data exposure. As Jardin learned, many more people may find that their medical records are filled with inaccuracies, mislabeled, or even misidentified.

The United States government is helping to lead the global charge to improve patients' access to their health data partly due to legislation passed during the height of the Great Recession: the HITECH Act of 2009. The Act provides hospitals, health providers, and others with a range of financial incentives designed to encourage them to adopt electronic health records (EHRs). In addition, U.S. regulators established a range of criteria, better known as Meaningful Use, designed to ensure that EHRs meet certain basic standards, are secure, and are being used in ways that will positively influence patient care, public health, and more.

Meaningful Use is being implemented in three stages or phases. [212] From a data access perspective, Stage 2 is important because it requires hospitals, providers, and others using EHRs to provide a certain percentage of patients with increased access to their medical information. [213]

On the surface, the fact that patients will be able to request and receive their personal health data more easily may not appear groundbreaking. But the health system's shift in the United States (and globally, as explained earlier in this book) from analog to digital recordkeeping is a big deal. Traditionally, hospitals, health providers, and others have kept paper-based records. This is bad for many reasons, including:

- **Data is Hard to Access:** Patients can't easily transfer their health records when they change hospitals, physicians, and more
- **Care is Compromised:** If they can't see patients' complete medical records, doctors working in different hospitals or parts of the country will be operating with incomplete information, which makes care less efficient
- **Mistakes Are Compounded:** If patients' records are paper-based and difficult to access, it's easier for mistakes to go unnoticed, which could cause serious medical problems in the future, e.g., in cases where patients are given the wrong medicine or dose based on inaccurate information

EHRs: A Step Forward, But Far from Perfect

While EHRs are viewed as superior to paper records, they are not without problems. One major issue is data accuracy. In an interview conducted for this book, patient advocate Dave deBronkart (or ePatient Dave) spoke at length about why he feels inaccurate health data deserves greater attention. In several instances, deBronkart has had to correct his (or others') medical records, including when he was misidentified as a woman in a critical chest x-ray.

deBronkart feels that if electronic health records are not checked for accuracy, patients and others adopting EHRs (and technologies leveraging EHR data) may lose confidence in them; however, he also feels issues associated with accuracy could be mitigated if patients (who he considers "one of the most undervalued resources" in the health system) are allowed to play a greater role in vetting and maintaining their personal medical records.

Another major issue with EHRs is that they may be exacerbating the very problem they were meant to solve: siloed health information. According to a 2013 Reuters report, "Many electronic health record systems do not coordinate with each other." This means that doctors still cannot easily access medical information about a patient who was initially treated in another hospital using a different EHR system. [214]

Despite the problems associated with EHRs, the fact remains that the benefits outweigh the negatives. This is important at a fundamental level because patients, caregivers, and medical professionals alike need access to health information in order to make better care-related decisions; however, having access to information is far from enough.

CareHacking is Not Just About Accessing Health Data, But Using It Effectively

While CareHacking, Jardin did much more than identify inaccuracies in her medical record; she *used* her health data to actively guide her care. In one case, Jardin's doctor told her that because a critical body scan was not yet available, her appointment would be delayed. Jardin promptly provided her latest scans, which she routinely requested, and even helped the doctor access her records. [215]

Jardin's self-advocacy demonstrates this important point: health data is only valuable when it is used to make an impact. Some patients—either because of their cultural background, temperament, health literacy level, or another reason—are not comfortable asking for or using their health data. In fact, this gap between patient knowledge and self-activation has been well documented in health for some time. The Patient Activation Measure (PAM), developed by Judy Hibbard and her colleagues at the University of Oregon, is a tool patients (and health providers) can use to determine their level of knowledge, skills, and willingness to manage their own health. [216] As patients achieve higher PAM scores, they progress from passively receiving care to engaging in new health behaviors.

Tools like PAM can answer the critical question of whether patients are willing and able to use health data delivered via EHRs and otherwise. The health and medical community can also use this information to support patients and help more of them feel comfortable with using health data to guide their health and medical care.

We have to emphasize one important point, however. Although many patients may not be ready to participate in all aspects of their care, we shouldn't assume most people would be unwilling to—especially in cases where they choose to seek help from a doctor. As Steve Wilkins, patient engagement expert, argued in a September 2012 post on his blog *Mind the Gap:* "[B]y definition, people who show up for a doctor's appointment are already engaged [in their care]." This is because their concerns, previous research, conversations with friends and family, and other pre-appointment activities suggest they are very interested in engaging with physicians and other providers. [217]

So far we have discussed the potential value as well as current issues with electronic health records, and examined the important question of patients' willingness to fully engage in their own care. Now we turn our attention to addressing whether support and information available via the Internet has accelerated patients' and caregivers' ability to improve their health and wellbeing.

Beyond Information: How Web-Powered CareHacking Has Improved ePatients' Health Management Abilities

Over the past decade or so, one of the most persistent questions people have had about the Internet is whether ubiquitous access to unverified or misleading content is harmful. The Pew Research Center addressed this question back in 2011 and found that 30% of U.S. adults "say they or someone they know has been helped by following medical advice or health information found online." [218]

Although Pew's finding illustrates that people are finding valuable information online, there is still a lot of concern about the overall quality of Web-health content. Doctors worry patients could be harmed by misinformation delivered by Dr. Google. Researchers complain about the lack of unbiased or correctly interpreted health information published on popular sites such as Wikipedia and Yahoo!. And global media sometimes presents overly simplistic conclusions from complex research in ways that can encourage false and unproven generalizations.

We know using the Web for education, to navigate loopholes, and get better, lower cost, and faster care is a core CareHacking activity. Although some still have questions about whether the Internet is largely valuable or harmful, we have learned that ePatients—especially caregivers—find it to be immensely helpful in a critical area: managing their health.

In the 2013 edition of digihealth pulse, Enspektos asked ePatients to rate whether the Web has improved their ability to talk with doctors, find affordable health care, get treatment faster, understand medications, or improve other aspects of their (or their family's care).[21]

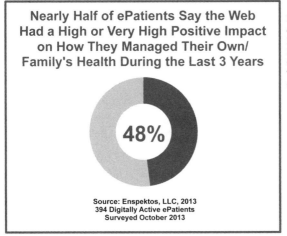

Nearly Half of ePatients Say the Web Had a High or Very High Positive Impact on How They Managed Their Own/ Family's Health During the Last 3 Years

48%

Source: Enspektos, LLC, 2013
394 Digitally Active ePatients
Surveyed October 2013

Figure XX: Percentage of ePatients Who Say Web Helped to Highly or Very Highly Improve Their Ability to Manage Their Own (or Their Family's) Care During the Past Three Years

Figure XXI: Percentage of ePatients Who Say Web Helped to Highly or
Very Highly Improve Their Ability to Manage Their Own (or Their Family's)
Care During the Past Three Years (by Caregiving Status)

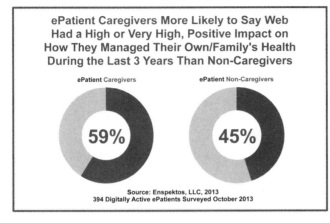

ePatient Caregivers More Likely to Say Web Had a High or Very High, Positive Impact on How They Managed Their Own/Family's Health During the Last 3 Years Than Non-Caregivers

ePatient Caregivers | ePatient Non-Caregivers

59% | 45%

Source: Enspektos, LLC, 2013
394 Digitally Active ePatients Surveyed October 2013

ePatients were also asked to think back about their experiences over the past three years and use a five-point rating scale to evaluate the Web's impact on their health management efforts (1 = No Improvement; 3 = Moderate Improvement; 5 = Very High Improvement).[22]

Enspektos learned that nearly half of ePatients say the Web had a high or very high, positive influence on their ability to manage their own, or family's care (Figure XX).

Enspektos also looked at how caregivers compared to non-caregivers. Overall, caregivers were much more likely to say the Web had a positive impact than non-caregivers (Figure XXI).

This data is yet another testament to the positive role the Web is playing in how people manage their health and wellbeing. Faced with increasing financial, medical, and societal pressures to become active stewards of their own care, ePatients are using the Web to hack the health system and benefit from the knowledge it contains.

Stories: CareHacking

The Blue Button Initiative: Giving Patients and Caregivers Immediate Access to Health Data

In 2010, the U.S. government launched a project designed to help Americans access their health data literally at the click of a virtual button. U.S. Chief Technology Officer Todd Park described the initial effort in 2011 as a "really simple initiative where Medicare beneficiaries, veterans, and military health beneficiaries all have secure Web sites where they can log on and look at their own data." [210] Users of health services provided by the U.S. government can click a blue button on secure federal sites to view and download their personal health information. Park and other officials did not anticipate having so many people interested in their health data and that Blue Button would become a nationwide movement that has spread to the private sector. To date, more than one million veterans of the U.S. armed forces have used the Blue Button to access their data. In addition, about 450 private and public sector organizations have pledged to make health data available to patients using Blue-Button technology via health providers, labs, insurance companies, and more. [219]

While Blue Button has had some early success, there is much room for improvement. Critically, more patients need to be informed about the program and understand what Blue Button can do for them. In addition, raw data delivered via the button is less than understandable and actionable. [220] In an effort to address some of these concerns, the U.S. government announced a program that will launch in 2014 designed to improve awareness of Blue Button and make health data it delivers easier to access and use. [221]

Learn More:

http://www.healthit.gov/patients-families/blue-button/about-blue-button

ZocDoc is Making Finding, Meeting, and Rating Doctors Easy

Back in 2007, a pioneering startup called ZocDoc took a concept that was already becoming commonplace in the services industry and applied it to the world of medicine. As consumers were becoming used to the ability to book a table at a restaurant and manage their meetings and calendars online, ZocDoc was making it easier for patients to see their doctors. ZocDoc was also helping people search for doctors based on region, insurance coverage, and quality—as rated by others.

ZocDoc was among the first of a growing number of companies working to help patients hack the system and easily find the best doctors, schedule appointments, and more. By early 2013, more than four million users from 2,000 cities had used the service per month. ZocDoc is one of the most successful and profitable startups helping consumers access better care quickly and efficiently.

Learn More: https://www.zocdoc.com

GoFundMe: Helping People Manage the High Costs of Medical Care

At the beginning of the book, we discussed the spiraling costs of health care in the United States and some parts of the world. In addition, consumers are being asked to assume greater financial responsibility for their medical expenses. As a result, some are turning to sites like Go-FundMe for help. People from around the world are using GoFundMe to launch and manage fundraising campaigns for those with a variety of illnesses, often collecting tens of thousands of dollars in the process.

GoFundMe represents a variation of a trend Rohit identified in his 2013 Annual Business Trend Report: "MeSourcing." However, no matter what you call it, people are using GoFundMe to make emotional appeals to others to help offset medical expenses for friends, family, and colleagues.

Learn More: http://www.gofundme.com/

---

[21] See Appendix I for more information about digihealth pulse.

[22] Percentage of ePatients selecting options 4 and 5 shown in Figures XX and XXI.

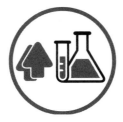

Trend 15:
Accelerated Trial-Sourcing

*Consumers with chronic diseases and other conditions are pioneering
the Accelerated Trial-Sourcing movement as they use digital tools to find
one another, complete the first stage of discovery to prepare for a clinical
study in real time, and recruit/entice the right pharmaceutical firms or
other researchers to conduct the research.*

Students arriving for the first day of classes at Harvard Medical School in the
fall of 1988 were about to get an unexpected greeting. Prepared to meet their
professors and fellow future physicians, they were instead surprised to encounter a group of protesters from the Boston Arm of ACT UP (the AIDS Coalition
to Unleash Power). In his book *Impure Science: AIDS Activism, and the Politics
of Knowledge,* author Steven Epstein described the scene:

> "While some of the demonstrators poured fake blood on the sidewalk,
> others presented the medical students with a mock 'course outline' for
> an 'AIDS 101' class . . . [that] listed discussion topics like . . . Medical
> elitism—Is the pursuit of elegant science leading to the destruction of
> our community?" [222]

In his analysis of the ACT UP protest, Epstein seized on the term "elegant science" as vitally important. Epstein suggested that it captures the essence of what the AIDS protesters were fighting against: the idea that medical research should be slowly conducted by experts far removed from the social, political, and human impact of their work. [222]

The ACT UP movement coined the picket-sign worthy tagline Silence = Death. During their 1988 protest, the Boston chapter of the group extended this concept by arguing that Elegant Science = Death. The protest was an inevitable product of its time. In the late 1980s, there were no effective treatments for the millions infected with HIV. Finding treatments was an urgent necessity. The traditional method of slow, careful, elegant medical research simply wasn't an option for those facing certain death.

In some respects the Accelerated Trial-Sourcing trend taking shape today has its roots in the AIDS protests of the 1980s and 1990s. Accelerated Trial-Sourcing is characterized by patients conducting their own experiments or self-reporting their reactions to prescribed treatments in order to help researchers more quickly and definitively determine the real-world effectiveness of treatments. This trend is the expression of the empowered and engaged patient who:

- Takes responsibility for reporting their own medical results
- Uses networks and data to actively recruit researchers from the private and public sectors and influences them to accelerate clinical studies.

It is clear that Accelerated Trial-Sourcing flows out of the patient power movement (initially inspired and fueled by AIDS activists in the 80s) that greatly influenced private and public sector research and funding across a range of conditions and diseases. The movement also shifted the balance of power between patients and scientists. [223] In a review of *Impure Science*, published in the *New York Times Magazine* in 1997, Jeffrey Goldberg described the immense impact of the AIDS protests this way:

"[AIDS protest groups] are infamous for outrageous street theater, but their real impact has been in the way in which they've influenced the scientific process. This influence—unimaginable in an earlier age, before the feminist health movement of the 1970s began questioning the omniscience of white men in white coats—is seen in manifold changes: in the way the National Institutes of Health organizes clinical studies, in the way pharmaceutical companies manufacture drugs, and in the way the F.D.A. speeds drugs through the approval process." [224]

AIDS activists and patients also thrust patient-led and inspired research, which is central to Accelerated Trial-Sourcing, onto the public stage. The 2012 film, *How to Survive a Plague*, documents the rise of "underground" drug trials. [225] In these studies, patients, with the assistance of medical researchers, tested unapproved drugs to determine whether they would prove effective against HIV.

For example, during the spring of 1989, scientists and researchers in Florida, New York, and California launched unsanctioned tests of Compound Q, which appeared to show promise against the disease. The trial, which was not approved by pharmaceutical companies or the Food and Drug Administration, was initiated partly out of concern that thousands of people were taking the experimental drug without supervision. [226] Compound Q was just one of the many medications patients turned to (and tested) in desperation in the era before effective AIDS treatments were approved by the Food and Drug Administration.

In the end, Accelerated Trial-Sourcing (like the AIDS movement before it) is all about patients fighting against the notion they have no say in medical research and that slow elegant science is the optimal way to bring new therapies to market. The difference between then and now comes down to how rapidly these efforts can be coordinated globally and the results can be shared immediately, thanks to the range of digital technologies and social networking tools that were largely unavailable decades ago.

Using Digital Technologies and Online Communities to Combat Elegant Science

During the 1980s, many activists with HIV acted out of desperation because their time was short. Today, many in the Accelerated Trial-Sourcing movement are motivated by a similar sense of urgency, especially people with amyotrophic lateral sclerosis (ALS), or Lou Gehrig's disease. There is no cure for ALS and current treatments are, at best, only partially effective. This is why a group of ALS patients used the Internet, social networks, and data analysis tools to conduct their own test of a home-brewed experimental drug. In 2012, ALS patient Ben Harris told the *Wall Street Journal*: "We simply don't have time to wait for the results of [clinical trials]. Our life spans are much shorter than the [Food and Drug Administration] approval process." [227]

The drug Harris and others were taking was a version of NP001, a medication developed by Neuraltus Pharmaceuticals. [228] Unable to enroll in an early NP001 trial, patients scoured patent filings, medical research, and other documents. They eventually came to believe NP001's main ingredient was sodium chlorite, which was available online at a low cost. After a year of debate and discussion, which took place largely in online patient forums, a group of ALS patients decided taking sodium chlorite was worth the risk. [228]

In the case of sodium chlorite, self-reported data from those taking the chemical suggested it was benefiting some patients; however, researchers from PatientsLikeMe disagreed. After examining data on sodium chlorite's effectiveness collected via the platform, PatientsLikeMe concluded it was ineffective and may even worsen some patients' ALS. [228]

There is a long tradition of patient-led research in the ALS community. And PatientsLikeMe (founded by two brothers who were inspired by their late third brother who suffered from ALS) is a social network that enables patients to share and analyze data on treatments for ALS, depression, and other diseases.

Patient-led research is not the only form of Accelerated Trial-Sourcing. In some cases, patients are having a say about which studies receive funding and voluntarily providing data and biologic material (such as DNA) to aid research.

For example, Tenovus, a cancer charity based in the United Kingdom, has formed a patient advisory council that has a significant influence on the non-profit's decisions about the studies it funds. [229] Another example is the Personal Genome Project. Launched in 2005, the project is a global network that uses publicly available, patient-provided genetic and ancestral data to accelerate genomic research. [230]

What all of these examples point to is the fundamental shift in how patient empowerment is driving more speed in the traditionally deliberate and "elegant" practice of medical research; yet, there is a predictable problem associated with this quest for speed: accuracy.

Why the Medical Community is Concerned About the Rise of Accelerated Trial-Sourcing

When underground AIDS drug trials took place in the late 1980s, many expressed concerns about these studies that are now being echoed by some who are wary of taking too much of a "real-time" patient-driven approach to medical research. A few of these concerns are:

- The drugs people are taking electively may not truly be safe, as they are often not tested for purity by drug firms and the FDA
- The results from studies may not be trustworthy as patients may not have the facilities, knowledge, or capability to adhere to established scientific protocols
- Patient-led studies could actually harm (and potentially even delay) more established and traditional clinical trials by surfacing previously unknown drug side-effects or discourage patients from enrolling

As the Accelerated Trial-Sourcing movement grows, the number of medical professionals and researchers voicing these concerns may increase. Apart from the obvious concern that patients will unintentionally harm themselves, the key research question often raised is whether studies conducted outside of the medical clinic using tools developed by companies such as PatientsLikeMe can truly provide reliable data. [231] Another key related question is whether it is ethical to conduct studies without a sham, or placebo treatment, as self-reported patient data can be unreliable or biased. [228]

We predict that these concerns will not prevent the Accelerated Trial-Sourcing movement from progressing. The motivation and desire to help the process of medical research for patients and their families facing sickness and (often) certain death is an undeniably powerful force that will drive them to do almost anything to find, test, and advocate for treatments they believe may save lives.

Some of the evidence supporting this prediction is the rapid rise in "crowd-sourced health research" (which is related to our Accelerated Trial-Sourcing trend) over the past few years. Melanie Swan of the MS Futures Group refers to it "as a nexus of three contemporary trends:

1. Citizen science (non-professionally trained individuals conducting science-related activities);
2. Crowdsourcing (use of Web-based technologies to recruit project participants); and
3. Medicine 2.0 / Health 2.0 (active participation of individuals in their health care particularly using Web 2.0 technologies)" [232]

In her analysis of the medical literature and Google search results, Swan found:

"In 2011, 1,920,000 results were returned for a Google search of the terms 'crowd-sourcing and health'; in 2010 and 2009 the comparative figure was 669,000 and 318,000 respectively. In January 2012, the term 'crowdsourcing' in a PubMed search yielded 16 publications, 13 of which were published in 2011." [232]

One of the major drivers of the Accelerated Trial-Sourcing trend may be the nature of the patient-empowerment movement itself . . . and how it motivates patients and caregivers to become more educated about their disease and potential treatments for it. Thanks to their own research, some patients are skeptical about traditional medical studies and view new digital and social technologies as vital tools that can help them educate themselves, accelerate research, and engage experts on their own terms.

Finally, the growing ranks of medical researchers and companies sympathetic to patients will continue to refine and develop tools and technologies that aid collaboration and research. In fact, some, such as PatientLikeMe's Jamie Heywood, are more than willing to accept the benefits, drawbacks, and skepticism resulting from innovation. [228]

Stories: Accelerated Trial-Sourcing

PatientsLikeMe Launches the Next Era of Patient-Informed Research With its Open Health Exchange

Building on the initial success of its open-source crowdsourcing initiatives to help develop and test treatments for ALS, in August 2013 PatientsLikeMe announced its new Open Research Exchange (ORE), which is supported by a $1.9 million grant from the Robert Wood Johnson Foundation. According to a PatientsLikeMe press release, ORE was created "to help researchers design, test, and openly share new ways to measure diseases and health issues." Perhaps most importantly, patients will help direct ORE's work. The platform will leverage PatientsLikeMe's more than 200,000 members to research and shape its activities. Projects announced to date include the development of questionnaires to help physicians assess how they work with seriously ill patients and the creation of an instrument patients with high blood pressure can use to capture how they are doing between doctor visits.

Learn More:

http://arstechnica.com/science/2011/04/crowdsourcing-a-clinical-trial-to-treat-als/

http://news.patientslikeme.com/press-release/patientslikeme-selects-first-pilot-users-open-research-exchang

---

Transparency Life Sciences Works With Patients to Accelerate Drug Development and Design Clinical Trials

Promoting itself as the "world's first drug development company based on open innovation," Transparency Life Sciences (TLS) relies on the dual principles of crowdsourcing and mobile technology to reduce costs related to drug development while increasing the speed of medical research. According to TLS, "A key element of [its] approach is incorporating insights gathered from a global crowd into its clinical protocols using the company's Internet-based Protocol Builder, an online tool that elicits input from patients, physicians, and researchers to help design clinical trials more efficiently and with greater relevance to clinical practice and patients' needs."

Learn More:

http://transparencyls.com/how-it-works

http://www.prnewswire.com/news-releases/fda-clears-ind-for-first-clinical-trial-protocol-developed-using-crowdsourcing-183922651.html

Conclusion:
How to Prepare for the Future of Health Care

As 2010 came to a close, more than 60 critics listed one extraordinary work of historical fiction as being among the best of the year. The book entitled *The Immortal Life of Henrietta* Lacks told the amazing story of a woman known only to most medical researchers as HeLa, but whose cancer cells had become one of the most important tools in medicine. [233] Taken without her knowledge in 1951, Lacks' cervical cancer tumor cells eventually helped scientists over the next several decades develop numerous medical advancements, including the polio vaccine, cloning, gene mapping, and in-vitro fertilization.

Around the same time that the cells of a poor, black, tobacco-farming woman were starting their immortal journey, another unknown Australian teenager named James Harrison was repaying a debt. In the mid-1940s, he had lost a lung to metastasized pneumonia and was facing a certain death. Thanks to thirteen liters of transfusions and heroic medicine, he survived, and vowed that he would repay the favor and become a blood donor himself.

In 1954, after he had given many blood transfusions, researchers found that Harrison's blood included a rare antibody that could help treat an illness known as Rhesus disease (named after the protein it contains which is normally found in the blood of Rhesus monkeys). Rhesus disease causes a mother's immune system to attack a fetus's bloodstream if the mother does not have the Rh protein and the baby inherits it from the father. It was from Harrison's blood that scientists ultimately developed the Anti-D vaccine, which was used to protect fetuses with Rhesus disease.

In recounting Harrison's story in his book *Now I Know*, author Dan Lewis dubbed him "the man with the golden arm" thanks to his lifetime dedication to giving blood more than 1,000 times—and helping doctors create the vaccine that is estimated to have treated more than two million babies who would otherwise have had Rhesus disease. [234]

What draws us to the stories of Henrietta Lacks and James Harrison is how they both underscore the same fundamental point: world-changing events sometimes have modest beginnings.

In this book, we aimed to introduce you to a collection of transformative trends in health care that are just beginning to take shape and will accelerate over the next few years. Some may seem smaller now, while others may immediately seem poised for big growth and impact. Predicting the future is always a tricky business. Not even the smartest futurist could have predicted the global impact of a seemingly insignificant social tool like Twitter.

One of the underlying beliefs of this book is that the signs of the future are already here. Identifying trends that matter relies on the art and science of arranging the patterns of what is happening today into a story of where they will take us tomorrow. *Great trends aren't spotted—they are curated.*

So as we come to the end of this book, one of the biggest questions you may be asking yourself—whether you work in the healthcare industry or just happen to be an engaged observer, or are an ePatient yourself—is . . . what does it all mean and perhaps more importantly, what should you do differently as a result?

As we wrote this book, we imagined our audience to be broad and include patients, entrepreneurs, government officials, doctors, and others. With such a large group of sub-audiences, the implications of a book like this are intentionally far reaching. To discuss all the potential ideas that the trends may inspire could certainly take another book! We do, however, have some small pieces of advice and final thoughts with which we would love to leave you.

For patients (and those caring for them), our hope is that you might use this book as a guide for understanding the rapid changes happening in health and medical care and as a tool to play a supporting role in your own empowerment. If you're asked to participate in a wellness program in exchange for discounts on your health insurance premiums, you'll be prepared. If you see an advertisement for the latest wearable device, or personal genetic test, you'll have a good understanding of the benefits—and drawbacks—of these technologies. If you're being treated a bit differently when you're about to leave the hospital—e.g., your doctor wants to communicate with you more frequently—you'll have an insider's perspective on why your physician is being so attentive. Finally, and most importantly, we hope we've illustrated that it is imperative to use knowledge gained via the Web (and other sources) to improve your and your family's overall health, and the care you receive.

For health providers, entrepreneurs, government officials, developers, marketers, students, and everyone else, we would like to leave you with two pieces of advice:

1. **Ask Bigger Questions:** It's easy to focus on the technology trend, study, or acquisition of the moment; yet, there is a big difference between knowledge and understanding. As we've seen, health can be a big, scary, expensive topic. We hope this book helps you think more deeply and to imagine bigger questions about the systems around us. It is not enough to simply watch what is happening in the moment. We need to ask ourselves why events are occurring and courageously pose bigger questions . . . which will then lead us to bigger answers.
2. **Remember the Ecosystem:** Solving the biggest challenges facing health and medical care will take a lot more than technology. Big solutions must bring the best of many worlds together. Shaping the future of health will require sensitivity and empathy, particularly being willing and able to walk in the shoes of others.

If there is one lesson we have learned through the process of writing and collecting the research and information in this book, it is this: people like us will drive health care's evolution. In a world filled with increasing technological solutions to problems, health care's future is not digital—it's human. And like you, we look forward to watching it unfold with hopeful optimism, clear-eyed realism, and continual awe.

A Final Request

If you enjoyed reading this book, we have one final request we would like to make of you—please share it with someone else! Ideas and facts can only spread if people know about them, and we appreciate every time anyone shares one of our ideas.

One of the most amazing benefits of being authors is having the opportunity to hear directly from readers about their experience reading this book. If you would like to e-mail us directly to share any thoughts about the book—we (Fard or Rohit) can be reached via the contact form located at www.epatient2015.com or directly at rohit@epatient2015.com OR fard@epatient2015.com.

Thanks for your help—and for reading this book.

For all press inquiries, comments, or just to get in touch, visit www.epatient2015.com and click the "Contact" link at the top of the page.

Official Book Web site: www.epatient2015.com
Official Book Twitter: @epatient2015

Appendix I:
About the digihealth pulse Research Methodology

Launched by Enspektos in 2012, digihealth pulse is an ongoing study designed to improve understanding of:

- How ePatients perceive and use a range of existing and emerging digital health technologies, such as wearable devices (e.g., Google Glass), mobile health applications, and social media tools
- Whether ePatients' perceptions and behaviors (e.g., opinion of Obamacare, willingness to get a flu vaccination) changed after viewing health content on Web sites like WebMD and social media sites such as Facebook and Twitter

The first question some may ask about digihealth pulse is: Why study ePatients? Why not conduct research with the general U.S. adult population? Some of the most important reasons Enspektos decided to focus on ePatients include:

- ePatients can provide important clues about how people will regard and use health technologies in the future.
- As discussed in this book, ePatients have become a force in the health landscape and are helping to reshape how we think about medical research, caregiving, and more. This is why it is important to gather as much information as possible about this group of people.
- ePatients are comfortable with a range of technologies and will be more likely to provide informed responses about, or have experience with, important

tools such as personal genomics, self-tracking devices, and more.

How Enspektos Defined ePatients and Ensured the Statistical Reliability of the Study Results

When Enspektos was planning digihealth pulse in early 2012, it looked carefully at data published by the Pew Research Center on the demographic characteristics of people who fit the following criteria: [235]

- Active online users (those telling Pew they used the Web yesterday)
- Users of social media sites such as Twitter and Facebook
- Individuals who used the Web to search for information (for themselves or someone else) on any health topic tracked by Pew (people who conduct online health searches are considered ePatients)

Enspektos used Pew's data to build a population (or sample) of approximately 400 ePatients matching the online habits described above and key demographic characteristics (i.e., age, gender, and race) of this group.[23] It was important for Enspektos to look at Web and social media use because it tracks ePatients' activities on these platforms.

In addition, because the ePatient population is typically more affluent and less racially diverse, Enspektos recruited more African American, Hispanic, and low-income individuals (statisticians call this "over sampling") to aid analysis of topics of special relevance to these groups.

As a point of comparison, organizations like Gallup typically survey about 1,000 Americans for polls about presidential elections. Enspektos recruited a larger number of people representing a smaller group of U.S. adults (ePatients) for its research.

How Enspektos Conducted digihealth pulse

digihealth pulse studies are conducted in two stages:

- Stage I – Survey: During each study, ePatients answered more than 70 survey questions about how they use and perceive digital technologies, their digital health activities (such as whether they ever sought personal genetic testing), caregiving, health status, and more.
- Stage II – Tracking: After completing the survey, ePatients agreed to have their online and social media activities tracked using a patent-pending technology developed by Enspektos called enmoebius. This digital surveillance and behavioral measurement platform provides real-time data on:
  - The types of Web and social media sites ePatients visit and content published on these platforms
  - Their activities on social sites (e.g., what they post and read)
  - How ePatients respond (in real time) to content published on these sites (e.g., whether their opinion of Obamacare changed after reading an article in the *New York Times* or if they decided to get a flu shot after seeing a Facebook post about influenza)

Survey data from two digihealth pulse studies conducted by Enspektos in 2012 and 2013 is included in this book. Wave I of digihealth pulse was launched in September 2012 and Wave II in October 2013, partly to capture data related to the launch of the health insurance-exchanges required by the U.S. Affordable Care Act.

For additional information about digihealth pulse, please visit: www.digihealth-pulse.info. To learn more about enmoebius, please visit: www.enspektos.com/enmoebius.

---

[23] Enspektos recruited a demographically representative group of 398 ePatients in 2012 and 394 in 2013.

Appendix II:
Resources and Further Reading

In *ePatient 2015*, we highlight a wide range of trends and technologies influencing health care. In our research process, we read hundreds of articles, dozens of research reports, and more than 15 books on the past, present, and future of health care.

In an effort to share our resources, all of the data in the book has been carefully annotated with references to sources. In addition to the endnotes provided in the book, we have created a collection of resources and further reading that we are publishing online to share with you.

At the Web site below, you will find a list of those resources, direct links to relevant materials, suggestions for great books we recommend, and our newsletter, which you can join to receive additional commentary about the trends featured in this book.

www.epatient2015.com

In addition to those resources, we would also like to offer you direct access to the original research behind the book (and much more) via Enspektos' digital health intelligence and advisory service, enmoebius bronze. Here are details on how you can access enmoebius bronze.

enmoebius bronze:
Future-Focused Digital Health Intelligence,
Insights and Advice from Enspektos

enmoebius bronze, which is powered by Enspektos, is a member-supported intelligence service featuring more than 250 reports, webinars, infographics, and more on the evolving digital health landscape. In November 2013, Enspektos began publishing content to the service, featuring additional insights on topics covered in *ePatient 2015* and analysis of digihealth pulse data not featured in this book.
In addition, enmoebius bronze members have exclusive access to insights and advice from digital health experts (including Fard Johnmar).

If you're interested in diving deeper into the themes, trends, and data discussed in *ePatient 2015*, join subscribers from top organizations like the Mayo Clinic on enmoebius bronze. Use the discount code EPATIENT15READER at registration to take 15% off your monthly or annual subscription fee. To learn more about how the service can help you and how to start your free 10-day trial, please visit:

http://digihealth.info/digihealthintel.

References

1. Anonymous. *Digital Health*. 2013 August 5 [cited 2013 August 23]; Available from: http://en.wikipedia.org/wiki/Digital_health.
2. Holliday, R. *The Walking Gallery*. 2011 April 30 [cited 2013 September 16]; Available from: http://reginaholliday.blogspot.com/2011/04/walking-gallery.html.
3. Rainie, L. and S. Fox, *The Online Health Care Revolution: How the Web Helps Americans Take Better Care of Themselves*. 2000, Pew Research Center: Washington, DC.
4. Ferguson, T., Health Online: How to Find Health Information, Support Groups, and Self-Help Communities in Cyberspace. 1995, Reading: Addison-Wesley/Perseus Books.
5. Ferguson, T., e-Patient Scholars Working Group, *e-Patients: How They Can Help Us Heal Healthcare*. 2007, Robert Wood Johnson Foundation
6. Fox, S. *E-patients, Cyberchondriacs, and Why We Should Stop Calling Names*. 2010 August 30 [cited 2013 August 18]; Available from: http://www.pewinternet.org/Commentary/2010/August/Epatients-Cyberchondriacs.aspx.
7. Fox, S., *Mobile Health 2012*. 2012, Pew Research Center: Washington, DC.
8. Anonymous. *Scanadu: Sending Your Smart Phone to Med School*. 2013 [cited 2013 April 20]; Available from: http://www.scanadu.com/.
9. Haig, S. *When the Patient is a Googler*. TIME Magazine, November 8 2007.
10. Meisel, Z.F. *Googling Symptoms Helps Patients and Doctors*. TIME Magazine January 19, 2011.
11. Johnson, D., A *$42 Million Gift Aims at Improving Bedside Manner*, in *New York Times* September 22, 2011: New York.

12. Fox, S. and M. Duggan, *Health Online 2013*. 2013, Pew Research Center: Washington, DC.
13. Anonymous, *Digital Health Funding Mid-Year Update*. 2013, Rock Health: San Francisco.
14. Anonymous. *Health 2.0 and Enspektos, LLC Talk Big Picture Health Technology Insights, the Future of Consumer Digital Health and More.* [Slide Presentation] 2013 [cited 2013 August 25]; Available from: http://www.slideshare.net/fjohnmar/big-picture-health-tch.
15. Anonymous, *Next Time, What Say We Boil a Consultant*, in *Fast Company* October 31, 1995.
16. Rosenthal, E., *American Way of Birth, Costliest in the World*. June 30, 2013, New York Times.
17. Anonymous, *The Cost of Having a Baby in the United States*. 2013, Truven Health Analytics.
18. Healy, M. *Senior Health Care Crisis Looms; Report Ranks States*. USA Today, May 28, 2013.
19. Marshall, S., K.M. McGarry, and J.S. Skinner, *The Risk of Out-of-Pocket Health Care Expenditure at End of Life*. NBER Working Paper, July 2010 (16170).
20. Laney, D., *3D Data Management: Controlling Data Volume, Velocity and Variety*. Application Delivery Strategies, 2001.
21. Siegel, E., *Predictive Analytics: The Power to Predict Who Will Click, Buy, Lie, or Die* 2013, Hoboken: John Wiley & Sons.
22. McBride, R. *10 Startups Fueling Pharma in Social Media*. FierceBiotechIT, June 17, 2013.
23. Rosner, D., *A Once Charitable Enterprise: Hospitals and Health Care in Brooklyn and New York, 1885-1915* 1st ed. 1982, Cambridge: Cambridge University Press.
24. Rosen, G., *The Structure of American Medical Practice, 1875-1941*. 1983, Philadelphia: University of Pennsylvania Press.
25. Eddy, D.M., *Evidence-Based Medicine: A Unified Approach*. Health Affairs, 2005. 24(1): p. 9-17.
26. Schiebinger, L., *Women's Health and Clinical Trials*. Journal of Clinical Investigation, 2003. 112(7): p. 973–977.
27. Yasuda, S.U., L. Zhang, and S.M. Huang, *The Role of Ethnicity in Variability in Response to Drugs: Focus on Clinical Pharmacology Studies*. Clinical Pharmacology and Therapeutics, 2008. 84(3): p. 417-423.
28. Ma, Q. and A.Y.H. Lu, *Pharmacogenetics, Pharmacogenomics, and Individualized Medicine*. Pharmacological Reviews, 2011. 63(2): p. 437-459.

29. Chen, P.W., *For New Doctors, 8 Minutes Per Patient* in *New York Times*. May 30, 2013.

30. Duncan, D.E., et al., *The Personalized Health Project: Identifying the Gaps Between Discovery and Application in the Life Sciences, and Proposed Solutions*. 2011, Ewing Marion Kauffman Foundation: Kansas City.

31. Anonymous. *PatientsLikeMe Research*. 2013 [cited 2013 August 20, 2013]; Available from: http://news.patientslikeme.com/research.

32. Topol, E., *The Creative Destruction of Medicine: How the Digital Revolution Will Create Better Health Care* 2012, New York: Basic Books.

33. Fogg, B.J., *Persuasive Technology: Using Computers to Change What We Think and Do* 2003, San Francisco: Morgan Kaufmann Publishers.

34. Sarasohn-Kahn, J., *Making Sense of Sensors: How New Technologies Can Change Patient Care*. 2013, California Healthcare Foundation: Oakland.

35. Anonymous. *Augmented Reality*. 2013 August 27, 2013 [cited 2013 August 27]; Available from: http://en.wikipedia.org/wiki/Augmented_reality.

36. Dooley, R., *Brainfluence : 100 Ways to Persuade and Convince Consumers with Neuromarketing* 2012, Hoboken: Wiley.

37. Burns, M. *Study: More Consumers Turn to Social Media for Health Research*. PharmaLive 2013 [cited 2013 October 11]; Available from: http://www.pharmalive.com/study-more-consumers-turn-to-social-media-for-health-research?cid=nl.phrm03.

38. Goyer, A. *Building Your Caregiving Team*. 2013 August 12 [cited 2013 August 29]; Available from: http://blog.aarp.org/2013/08/12/amy-goyer-find-help-for-caregiver/.

39. Fox, S., *Family Caregivers Online*. 2012, Pew Research Center: Washington, DC.

40. Anonymous. *Family Caregivers Are Wired for Health*. 2013 June 20 [cited 2013 August 29]; Available from: http://www.pewinternet.org/Press-Releases/2013/Family-Caregivers-are-Wired-for-Health.aspx.

41. Goyer, A. *The Dementia Tsunami is Headed Your Way*. 2013 March 10 [cited 2013 August 29, 2013]; Available from: http://blog.tedmed.com/?p=2858.

42. Fox, S. *Peer-to-Peer Health Care is a Slow Idea That Will Change the World*. 2013 August 3 [cited 2013 August 29]; Available from: http://susannahfox.com/2013/08/03/peer-to-peer-health-care-is-a-slow-idea-that-will-change-the-world/.

43. Fox, S., *Peer-to-Peer Health Care*. 2011, Pew Research Center: Washington, DC.

44. Fox, S. and K. Purcell, *Chronic Disease and the Internet*. 2010, Pew

Research Center: Washington, DC.

45. Comstock, J. *VA Launches Caregiver Pilot with 10 New Apps.* MobiHealthNews, 2013.

46. Anonymous *More Doctors Starting to Prescribe Mobile Apps for Chronic Conditions.* iHealth Beat, April 2, 2013.

47. Anonymous. *Innovator Chat: How Watson Can Transform Healthcare.* 2013 April 22 [cited 2013 September 1]; Available from: http://www.theatlantic.com/sponsored/ibm-watson/archive/2013/04/innovator-chat-how-watson-can-transform-healthcare/274584/.

48. Guizzo, E., *Hiroshi Ishiguro: The Man Who Made a Copy of Himself,* in *IEEE Spectrum* April 23, 2010.

49. Lim, A. *Japanese Robot Actroid Gets More Social, Has No Fear of Crowds.* 2013 March 13 [cited 2013 August 20, 2013]; Available from: http://spectrum.ieee.org/automaton/robotics/humanoids/japanese-robot-actroid-sit.

50. Anonymous, *The Patient Protection and Affordable Care Act.* 2010: United States government. p. 290.

51. Rau, J., *Hospitals Face Pressure to Avert Readmissions,* in *New York Times* November 26, 2012: New York.

52. Anonymous. *Readmissions Reduction Program.* 2012 [cited 2013 September 1]; Available from: http://cms.gov/Medicare/Medicare-Fee-for-Service-Payment/AcuteInpatientPPS/Readmissions-Reduction-Program.html/.

53. Boutwell, A. *Time to Get Serious About Hospital Readmissions.* October 10, 2012 [cited 2013 September 1, 2013]; Available from: http://healthaffairs.org/blog/2012/10/10/time-to-get-serious-about-hospital-readmissions/.

54. Rau, J. *Medicare Revises Hospitals' Readmissions Penalties* Kaiser Health News, October 2, 2012.

55. Rau, J. *Bigger Readmissions Fines Hit Hospitals* Health IT News, August 5, 2013.

56. Wenner, D., *Highmark Health Insurance Wants to Reduce Patient Readmissions to Hospitals,* in *The Patriot-News* July 16, 2012.

57. Hall, S. *Analytics Help Hospital Cut Readmissions by 25%.* Fierce Health IT, June 28, 2013.

58. Anonymous, *When IT Matters: Improving Care Delivery and Patient Outcomes through Technology* 2013, College of Healthcare Information Management Executives, El Camino Hospital: Ann Arbor, Michigan.

59. Anonymous. *The GiraffPlus Project.* 2013 [cited 2013 September 1]; Available from: http://www.giraffplus.eu/.

60. Anonymous, *In the Spotlight: The Affordable Care Act and Wellness Programs*. 2012, BlueCross BlueShield of North Carolina: Durham, North Carolina.

61. Anonymous, *Incentives for Nondiscriminatory Wellness Programs in Group Health Plans* D.o.t.T.E.B.S.A. Internal Revenue Service, Department of Labor; Centers for Medicare & Medicaid Services, Department of Health and Human Services, Editor. 2013: Washington, DC. p. 123.

62. Jost, T. *Implementing Health Reform: Workplace Wellness Programs*. May 29, 2013 [cited 2013 August 29]; Available from: http://healthaffairs.org/blog/2013/05/29/implementing-health-reform-workplace-wellness-programs/.

63. Mattke, S., et al., *Workplace Wellness Programs Study: Final Report*. 2013, RAND Health: Santa Monica, CA.

64. Dolan, B. *Humana Bought Healthrageous to Build Out Vitality*. 2013 October 7 [cited 2013 October 13]; Available from: http://mobihealthnews.com/26099/humana-bought-healthrageous-to-build-out-vitality/.

65. Anonymous. *About UX 2014*. 2012 [cited 2013 Sepember 24]; Available from: http://www.ux2014.org/about-ux-2014.

66. Condit, R. *Batteries Not Included: The Gaps of Enroll UX 2014*. 2012 November 2 [cited 2013 October 21]; Available from: Batteries Not Included: The Gaps of Enroll UX 2014.

67. Anonymous. *Summit on Healthcare Technology in Nonclinical Settings Opens with a Call for 'Empathy in Design'*. 2013 October 9, 2013 [cited 2013 October 25]; Available from: http://www.aami.org/news/2013/100913_Summit_on_Healthcare_Opens.html.

68. Sengupta, S., *What You Didn't Post, Facebook May Still Know*, in *New York Times* March 25, 2013.

69. Singer, N., *A Data Broker Offers a Peek Behind the Curtain*, in *New York Times* August 31, 2013: New York.

70. Anonymous. *What Is a "Covered Entity" Under HIPAA?* 2013 [cited 2013 August 15]; Available from: http://www.hrsa.gov/healthit/toolbox/HealthITAdoptiontoolbox/PrivacyandSecurity/entityhipaa.html.

71. Anonymous. *Press Release: New Rule Protects Patient Privacy, Secures Health Information*. January 17, 2013 [cited 2013 August 15]; Available from: http://www.hhs.gov/news/press/2013pres/01/20130117b.html.

72. Abrams, L., *Study: Facebook Likes Predict Obesity*, in *The Atlantic* April 29, 2013.

73. Chunara, R., et al., *Assessing the Online Social Environment for Surveillance of Obesity Prevalence*. PLOS ONE, 2013. 8(4): p. e61373.

74. Kosinski, M., D. Stillwell, and T. Graepel, *Private Traits and Attributes Are Predictable from Digital Records of Human Behavior.* Proceedings of the National Academy of Sciences, 2013.

75. Ackerman, L., *Mobile Health and Fitness Applications and Information Privacy: Report to California Consumer Protection Foundation.* 2013, Privacy Rights Clearinghouse: San Diego.

76. Anonymous. *Breaches Affecting 500 or More Individuals.* 2012 http://www. hhs.gov/ocr/privacy/hipaa/administrative/breachnotificationrule/ breachtool.html [cited 2013 August 13].

77. Dimick, C. *OCR Reports Over 21 Million Impacted by Large-Scale Breaches.* 2012 September 12 [cited 2013 August 13]; Available from: http://journal.ahima.org/2012/09/12/three-years-later-ocr-reports-over-21-million-impacted-by-large-scale-breaches/.

78. Wadhwa, T. *Yes, You Can Hack a Pacemaker (And Other Medical Devices Too).* 2012 December 6 [cited 2013 June 12]; Available from: http:// www.forbes.com/sites/singularity/2012/12/06/yes-you-can-hack-a-pacemaker-and-other-medical-devices-too/.

79. Talbot, D., *Computer Viruses Are "Rampant" on Medical Devices in Hospitals* in *MIT Technology Review* October 17, 2012.

80. Huesch, M.D., *Privacy Threats When Seeking Online Health Information.* JAMA Internal Medicine, 2013.

81. Madigan, L. *Information Request to WebMD.* 2013 July 11 [cited 2013 September 3]; Available from: http://illinoisattorneygeneral.gov/ pressroom/2013_07/Information_Request_to_WebMD.pdf.

82. Kane, Z.M. *Fitbit Users Are Unwittingly Sharing Details of Their Sex Lives with the World.* 2011 July 3 [cited 2013 March 22]; Available from: http://thenextweb.com/insider/2011/07/03/fitbit-users-are-inadvertently-sharing-details-of-their-sex-lives-with-the-world/.

83. Bryant, M. *Details of Fitbit Users' Sex Lives Removed from Search Engine Results* 2011 July 4 [cited 2013 March 22]; Available from: http:// thenextweb.com/insider/2011/07/04/details-of-fitbit-users-sex-lives-removed-from-search-engine-results/.

84. Anonymous, *Data Privacy Day Privacy Survey 2013.* 2013, Microsoft: Redmond.

85. Thompson, D. *Google's CEO: 'The Laws Are Written by Lobbyists'.* 2010 October 1 [cited 2013 August 21]; Available from: http://www. theatlantic.com/technology/archive/2010/10/googles-ceo-the-laws-are-written-by-lobbyists/63908/ - video.

86. Anderson, T.H., *Becoming Sane with Psychohistory.* Historian, 1978. **41**(1): p. 1 - 20.

87. Gross, T., *Interview with Issac Asimov,* in *Fresh Air* 1987, National Public

Radio.

88. Johnmar, F., *The Rise of Just-in-Time Health Information Systems.* 2013, Enspektos, LLC: New York.

89. Talbot, D., *Big Data from Cheap Phones,* in *MIT Technology Review* April 23, 2013.

90. Anonymous. *Ginger.io: The Science.* 2013 [cited 2013 March 31, 2013]; Available from: http://ginger.io/the-science/.

91. Anonymous, *To Err Is Human.* 1999, Institute of Medicine: Washington, DC.

92. Anonymous. *What Is Almere DataCapital?* 2013 [cited 2013 September 30]; Available from: http://www.almeredatacapital.nl/index. php?option=com_content&view=article&id=68&Itemid=255.

93. Hertsgaard, M., *Michelle Obama's Fresh Food Revolution,* in *The Nation* April 20, 2009.

94. Schlosser, E., *Fast Food Nation: The Dark Side of the All-American Meal.* 1st Mariner Books Edition ed. 2001, New York: Houghton Mifflin Harcourt.

95. Schlosser, E. *Still a Fast-Food Nation: Eric Schlosser Reflects on 10 Years Later.* 2012 May 12 [cited 2013 September 25]; Available from: http:// www.thedailybeast.com/articles/2012/03/12/still-a-fast-food-nation-eric-schlosser-reflects-on-10-years-later.html.

96. Appel, L.J., et al., *A Clinical Trial of the Effects of Dietary Patterns on Blood Pressure.* New England Journal of Medicine, 1997. **336**(16): p. 1117-1124.

97. Wallach, J.J., *How America Eats: A Social History of U.S. Food and Culture* 2013, Plymouth: Rowman and Littlefield Publishers.

98. Sinclair, U., *The Jungle* 1906: self-published.

99. Pollan, M., *The Food Movement, Rising,* in *The New York Review of Books* May 20, 2010 New York Review of Books New York.

100. Anonymous. *Meet the 'Always On' Consumer.* 2013 [cited 2013 October 28]; Available from: http://www.experian.co.uk/marketing-services/ always-on-consumer.html.

101. Reitz, C., et al., *Variants in the ATP-Binding Cassette Transporter (ABCA7), Apolipoprotein E œμ4, and the Risk of Late-Onset Alzheimer Disease in African Americans.* JAMA, 2013. **309**(14): p. 1483-1492.

102. Brin, S. *LRRK2.* 2008 September 18 [cited 2013 September 20]; Available from: http://too.blogspot.com/2008/09/lrrk2.html.

103. Goetz, T., *Sergey Brin's Search for a Parkinson's Cure,* in *Wired* July 2010.

104. Goetz, T., *The Decision Tree: Taking Control of Your Health in the New Era of Personalized Medicine* 2010, New York: Rodale.

105. Manolio, T.A., *Bringing Genome-Wide Association Findings into Clinical*

Use. Nature Reviews Genetics, 2013. **14**(8): p. 549-558.

106. Long, J., et al., *Evaluating Genome-Wide Association Study-Identified Breast Cancer Risk Variants in African-American Women.* PLOS ONE, 2013. 8(4): p. e58350.

107. Carlson, C.S., et al., *Generalization and Dilution of Association Results from European GWAS in Populations of Non-European Ancestry: The PAGE Study.* PLOS Biol, 2013. **11**(9): p. e1001661.

108. Anonymous. *Genotyping Technology.* 2010 [cited 2013 September 27]; Available from: https://http://www.23andme.com/more/genotyping/.

109. Khoury, M.J. *Think Before You Spit: Do Personal Genomic Tests Improve Health?* 2011 August 25 [cited 2013 September 27]; Available from: http://blogs.cdc.gov/genomics/2011/08/25/think-before-you-spit-do-personal-genomic-tests-improve-health/.

110. Proffitt, A. *Too Much to Ignore: Anne Wojcicki's Plan for Health Care and Big Data.* Bio-IT World May 23, 2013.

111. Zimmerman, E. *The Race to a $100 Genome* 2013 June 25 [cited 2013 September 14]; Available from: http://money.cnn.com/2013/06/25/technology/enterprise/low-cost-genome-sequencing/index.html.

112. Anonymous. *Cost per Genome.* 2013 [cited 2013 September 14]; Available from: http://www.genome.gov/images/content/cost_per_genome.jpg.

113. Jolie, A., *My Medical Choice* in *New York Times* 2013, New York Times.

114. Kepler, A.W. *Angelina Jolie's Aunt Dies of Breast Cancer.* 2013 May 27 [cited 2013 September 27]; Available from: http://artsbeat.blogs.nytimes.com/2013/05/27/angelina-jolies-aunt-dies-of-breast-cancer/?_r=0.

115. Neporent, L. *Angelina Jolie's Double Mastectomy Fueling National Debate.* 2013 June 4 [cited 2013 September 27]; Available from: http://abcnews.go.com/Health/angelina-jolies-double-mastectomy-fueling-national-debate/story?id=19315336.

116. Singer, E., *The Personal Genome Project,* in *MIT Technology Review* January 20, 2006.

117. Anonymous. *Personal Genome Project.* 2013 November 7 [cited 2013 November 7]; Available from: http://en.wikipedia.org/wiki/Personal_Genome_Project.

118. Anonymous, *Innocenti Report Card: A League Table of Child Deaths by Injury in Rich Nations.* 2001, UNICEF Innocenti Research Centre: Florence, Italy.

119. Lee, C., et al., *Effectiveness of Speed-Monitoring Displays in Speed Reduction in School Zones.* Transportation Research Record: Journal of the Transportation Research Board, 2006. **1973**(1): p. 27-35.

120. Goetz, T., *Harnessing the Power of Feedback Loops*, in *Wired* July 2011.

121. Anonymous, *Applying Behavioural Insight to Health* 2010, Cabinet Office Behavioural Insights Team.

122. Sunstein, C.R., *It's for Your Own Good!*, in *New York Review of Books* March 7, 2013: New York.

123. Sunstein, C.R., *Empirically Informed Regulation*. University of Chicago Law Review, 2011. 78: p. 1349-1429.

124. Swan, M., *The Quantified Self: Fundamental Disruption in Big Data Science and Biological Discovery*. Big Data, 2013. 1(2): p. 85-99.

125. Fox, S. and M. Duggan, *Tracking for Health*. 2013, Pew Research Center: Washington.

126. Carter M.C., et al., *Adherence to a Smartphone Application for Weight Loss Compared to Website and Paper Diary: Pilot Randomized Controlled Trial*. Journal of Medical Internet Research, 2013. 15(4): p. e32.

127. Anonymous. *CHART: Wearable Computing Market Estimates Are All Over the Place*. 2013 April 16 [cited 2013 May 20]; Available from: http://www.businessinsider.com/chart-wearable-computing-market-estimates-are-all-over-the-place-2013-4.

128. Ryan, L. *Why the Digital Health Industry is About to Fail*. 2013 October 11 [cited 2013 October 11]; Available from: http://blog.gethealthapp.com/post/63681783790/why-the-digital-health-industry-is-about-to-fail.

129. Lupton, D., *The Digitally Engaged Patient: Self-Monitoring and Self-Care in the Digital Health Era*. Social Theory & Health, 2013. 11(3): p. 256-270.

130. Solon, O. *Walter De Brouwer: We Want a 'Tricorder' to Replace the Thermometer*. 2013 October 17 [cited 2013 October 29]; Available from: http://www.wired.co.uk/news/archive/2013-10/17/walter-de-brouwer-scanadu.

131. Yohn, D.L. *Ten Commandments of Digital Health* 2012 July 2 [cited 2013 September 7]; Available from: http://deniseleeyohn.com/bites/2012/07/02/ten-commandments-of-digital-health/.

132. Anonymous. *Partnership to Fight Chronic Disease: 2013 Almanac of Chronic Disease*. 2013 September 10 [cited 2013 September 16]; Available from: http://almanac.fightchronicdisease.org/Home.

133. Bloom, D.E., et al., *The Global Economic Burden of Noncommunicable Diseases*. 2011, World Economic Forum: Geneva.

134. Anonymous, *Partnership to Fight Chronic Disease: 2008 Almanac of Chronic Disease*. 2008, Partnership to Fight Chronic Disease: Washington, DC.

135. Anonymous. *Relationship Between Poverty and Overweight or Obesity*.

2010 [cited 2013 August 26]; Available from: http://frac.org/initiatives/hunger-and-obesity/are-low-income-people-at-greater-risk-for-overweight-or-obesity/.

136. Anonymous, *Understanding the Impact of Health IT in Underserved Communities and Those with Health Disparities.* 2013, NORC at the University of Chicago; Office of the National Coordinator for Health Information Technology, Department of Health and Human Services: Washington, DC.

137. Anonymous, *2012 National Healthcare Quality and Disparities Report.* 2013, Agency for Healthcare Research and Quality, U.S. Department of Health and Human Services: Rockville.

138. Haseltine, W.A., *Affordable Excellence: The Singapore Healthcare Story—How to Create and Manage Sustainable Healthcare Systems* 2013, Washington, DC: Brookings Institution Press.

139. Duggan, M. and A. Smith, *Cell Internet Use 2013.* 2013, Pew Research Center: Washington, DC.

140. Anonymous. *Consumer Medical Devices Set for Stable Market Growth as Health Concerns Show No Sign of Ebbing* 2013 September 12 [cited 2013 September 25]; Available from: http://press.ihs.com/press-release/design-supply-chain-media/consumer-medical-devices-set-stable-market-growth-health-con.

141. Khalsa, A. *Why Israel is Poised to Soon Lead Medical Device Industry Growth.* 2013 September 9 [cited 2013 October 5]; Available from: http://marketrealist.com/2013/09/must-know-israel/.

142. Milian, M. *Do Black Tech Entrepreneurs Face Institutional Bias?* 2011 November 14 [cited 2013 September 10]; Available from: http://www.cnn.com/2011/11/11/tech/innovation/black-tech-entrepreneurs/index.html.

143. Arrington, M. *Oh Shit, I'm a Racist.* 2011 October 28 [cited 2013 September 10]; Available from: http://uncrunched.com/2011/10/28/oh-shit-im-a-racist/.

144. Williams, H. *A Modest Proposal: Thinking Outside the White Male Box.* 2013 June 11 [cited 2013 September 19]; Available from: http://www.huffingtonpost.com/hank-williams/a-modest-proposal-thinkin_b_3417950.html.

145. Anonymous. *Rock Report: Women in Health.* [SlideShare Presentation] 2012 [cited 2013 September 16]; Available from: http://rockhealth.com/resources/rock-reports/women-in-health/.

146. Horn, B.I. *Bringing Diversity to the Health Tech Ecosystem.* 2013 August 31 [cited 2013 September 20]; Available from: http://pulseandsignal.com/events/bringing-diversity-to-the-health-tech-ecosystem/ - more-

2220.
147. Jimison, H., et al., *Barriers and Drivers of Health Information Technology Use for the Elderly, Chronically Ill, and Underserved* 2008, Agency for Healthcare Research and Quality: Rockville.
148. Jenkins, H., et al., *Confronting the Challenges of Participatory Culture: Media Education for the 21st Century*. 2005, The MacArthur Foundation: Chicago.
149. Anhøj, J. and L. Nielsen, *Quantitative and Qualitative Usage Data of an Internet-Based Asthma Monitoring Tool.* Journal of Medical Internet Research, 2013. 6(3): p. e23.
150. Combs, V. *AARP Reality Check: Members Tell Healthcare Startups Which Ideas Are on Time.* 2013 July 12 [cited 2013 September 20]; Available from: http://medcitynews.com/2013/07/aarp-reality-check-members-tell-healthcare-startups-which-ideas-are-on-time/.
151. McCraw Crow, S. *Is Your Baby Growing Normally?* . [cited 2013 October 15]; Available from: http://www.parents.com/baby/development/problems/baby-growing-normally/.
152. Buettner, D., *The Blue Zones: Lessons for Living Longer from the People Who've Lived the Longest* 2008, Washington, DC: National Geographic Society.
153. McFarland, M., *WellBeing Toronto Promotes Neighborhood Vibrancy, Government Transparency and Open Data* in *Azavea Journal* August 4, 2011.
154. Perman, C. *The Most Walkable Cities in America*. 2011 April 19 [cited 2013 August 15]; Available from: http://www.cnbc.com/id/42668491.
155. Anonymous. *America Walks: Benefits of a Walkable Community*. 2008 [cited 2013 August 15]; Available from: http://americawalks.org/resources/benefitsofawalkablecommunity/.
156. Cortright, J., *Walking the Walk: How Walkability Raises Housing Values* 2009, CEOs for Cities: Chicago.
157. Anonymous, *2013 National Association of Realtors Home Buyer and Seller Generational Trends*. 2013, National Association of Realtors: Chicago, IL.
158. Keenan, T.A., *Home and Community Preferences of the 45+ Population*. 2010, AARP: Washington, DC.
159. Anonymous. *Methodology: Gallup-Healthways Well-Being Index*. 2008 [cited 2013 August 25]; Available from: http://www.well-beingindex.com/methodology.asp.
160. Anonymous. *About the Blue Zones Project*. 2013 [cited 2013 September 1]; Available from: https://http://www.bluezonesproject.com/about_bluezones_project.

161. Anonymous. *Blue Zones Certification.* 2013 [cited 2013 September 1]; Available from: https://http://www.bluezonesproject.com/communities/organization/certifications.

162. Harris, S. *English Pupils Two Years Behind Chinese in Maths by the Age of 16.* 2013 February 21 [cited 2013 August 15]; Available from: http://www.dailymail.co.uk/news/article-2282577/English-pupils-years-Chinese-maths-age-16.html - ixzz2k7Gxo4sV.

163. Hanushek, E.A., P.E. Peterson, and L. Woessmann, *U. S. Math Performance in Global Perspective: How Well Does Each State Do at Producing High-Achieving Students?* 2010, Harvard's Program on Education Policy and Governance; Education Next; Taubman Center for State and Local Government: Cambridge.

164. Khamsi, R. *Mother Tongue May Determine Maths Skills.* 2006 June [cited 2013 October 1]; Available from: http://web.archive.org/web/20060701210510/http://www.newscientist.com/article/dn9422-mother-tongue-may-determine-maths-skills.html.

165. Anonymous. *Human Brain Project: Overview.* 2013 [cited 2013 October 15]; Available from: https://http://www.humanbrainproject.eu/discover/the-community/overview.

166. Anonymous. *Remarks by the President on the BRAIN Initiative and American Innovation.* 2013 April 2 [cited 2013 July 23]; Available from: http://www.whitehouse.gov/the-press-office/2013/04/02/remarks-president-brain-initiative-and-american-innovation.

167. Clay, R.A., *Functional Magnetic Resonance Imaging: A New Research Tool.* 2007, American Psychological Association: Washington, DC.

168. Khamsi, R., *Brain Scans Could Become EKGs for Mental Disorders,* in *TIME Magazine* June 28, 2013.

169. Kubie, J. *What's Wrong with Neuroscience (fMRI)?* 2012 December 3 [cited 2013 September 12]; Available from: http://coronaradiata.net/2012/12/03/whats-wrong-with-neuroscience-fmri/.

170. Marcus, G., *Neuroscience Fiction,* in *The New Yorker* December 2, 2012.

171. Chow, D. *Brain-Mapping Project's Vision Coming into Focus.* 2013 May 14 [cited 2013 September 13]; Available from: http://www.livescience.com/31984-brain-mapping-project-planning.html.

172. Anonymous. *Brain Research through Advancing Innovative Neurotechnologies (BRAIN) Initiative.* 2013 [cited 2013 September 15]; Available from: http://www.nih.gov/science/brain/.

173. Anonymous. *Brain Imaging Studies: Study Overview.* 2010 [cited 2013 October 21]; Available from: http://eatingdisorders.ucsd.edu/research/imaging/.

174. Anonymous. *Brain-Mapping Increases Understanding of Alcohol's Effects*

on First-Year College Students. 2013 [cited 2013 August 21]; Available from: http://www.sciencedaily.com/releases/2013/03/130319124308. htm.

175. Anonymous. *Ask the Expert: How Do Neurofeedback and Brain Mapping Help Treat ADHD?* 2013 May 1 [cited 2013 August 1]; Available from: http://www.nymetroparents.com/article/neruofeedback-and-brain-mapping-in-diagnosing-and-treating-adhd.

176. Badger, E. *Corridors of the Mind: Could Neuroscientists Be the Next Great Architects?* 2012 November 5 [cited 2013 May 23]; Available from: http://www.psmag.com/culture/corridors-of-the-mind-49051/.

177. Isaacson, W., *Steve Jobs* 2011, New York: Simon and Schuster.

178. Amri, R. *Why Did Steve Jobs Choose Not to Effectively Treat His Cancer?* 2011 October 12 [cited 2013 September 22]; Available from: http://www.quora.com/Steve-Jobs/Why-did-Steve-Jobs-choose-not-to-effectively-treat-his-cancer.

179. Stoneman, P., et al., *Incommensurable Worldviews? Is Public Use of Complementary and Alternative Medicines Incompatible with Support for Science and Conventional Medicine?* PLOS ONE, 2013. 8(1): p. e53174.

180. Barnes, P.M., B. Bloom, and R.L. Nahin, *Complementary and Alternative Medicine Use among Adults and Children: United States. 2007.* 2008, Centers for Disease Control and Prevention: Atlanta.

181. Anonymous, *Complementary and Alternative Medicine: What People Aged 50 and Older Discuss with Their Health Care Providers* 2011, AARP and the National Center for Complementary and Alternative Medicine Washingtion, DC.

182. Wald, N.J., *Commentary: A Brief History of Folic Acid in the Prevention of Neural Tube Defects* International Journal of Epidemiology, 2011. 40(5): p. 1154-6.

183. Anonymous, *Complementary and Alternative Medicine in the United States.* 2005, National Academy of Sciences: Washington.

184. Anonymous, *Smart Prevention — Health Care Cost Savings Resulting from the Targeted Use of Dietary Supplements.* 2013, Council for Responsible Nutrition Foundation and Frost & Sullivan: Washington.

185. Anonymous. *NCCAM Third Strategic Plan: 2011–2015.* 2012 February 9 [cited 2013 September 18]; Available from: http://nccam.nih.gov/about/plans/2011.

186. Orenstein, B.W. *Is Dead Sea Salt an Effective Psoriasis Treatment?* 2013 March 29 [cited 2013 July 16]; Available from: http://www.everydayhealth.com/psoriasis/can-dead-sea-salt-treat-psoriasis.aspx.

187. Goldman, E. *Despite Recession, Natural Medicine Continues to Grow* 2012 May 24 [cited 2013 August 15]; Available from: http://www. holisticprimarycare.net/news/1336-despite-recession-natural-medicine-continues-to-grow.

188. Jurenk, J.S., *Anti-Inflammatory Properties of Curcumin, a Major Constituent of Curcuma longa: A Review of Preclinical and Clinical Research.* Alternative Medicine Review, 2009. **14**(2): p. 141-153.

189. Anonymous. *Tumeric.* 2013 [cited 2013 July 29]; Available from: http://www.whfoods.com/genpage.php?tname=foodspice&dbid=78.

190. Dennis, J. *2012 International Herb & Botanical Trends.* 2012 July 1 [cited 2013 July 9]; Available from: http://www.nutraceuticalsworld.com/issues/2012-07/view_features/2012-international-herb-botanical-trends/.

191. Anonymous. *Map: Prevalent U.S. Health Problems.* 2013 [cited 2013 October 15]; Available from: http://www.cnn.com/interactive/2011/11/health/health.map/.

192. Anonymous. *Bible Belt.* 2013 October 20 [cited 2013 October 20]; Available from: http://en.wikipedia.org/wiki/Bible_Belt.

193. Anonymous. *What Is the Daniel Plan?* [cited 2013 August 15]; Available from: http://www.danielplan.com/whatistheplan/.

194. de Botton, A., *Religion for Atheists: A Non-Believer's Guide to the Uses of Religion* 2012, New York: Pantheon Books.

195. Peckham, M. *The Inexorable Decline of World of Warcraft.* 2013 May 9 [cited 2013 October 9]; Available from: http://techland.time.com/2013/05/09/the-inexorable-decline-of-world-of-warcraft/.

196. Anonymous. *The Games for Health Project.* 2013 [cited 2013 October 9]; Available from: http://www.rwjf.org/en/grants/grantees/GamesforHealth.html.

197. Anonymous. *OptumizeMe.* 2010 [cited 2013 October 9]; Available from: http://www.uhc.com/innovation/2010_third_quarter/optumizeme.htm.

198. Alcorn, S. *Get a Discount on Health Care—If You Wear a Tracking Bracelet.* 2013 October 11 [cited 2013 October 11]; Available from: http://www.marketplace.org/topics/health-care/get-discount-health-care-if-you-wear-tracking-bracelet.

199. Hollindale, C. *Gamifying Your Health with Google Glass: A Glimpse into the Future.* 2013 May 2 [cited 2013 October 7]; Available from: http://venturebeat.com/2013/05/02/gamifying-your-health-with-google-glass-a-glimpse-into-the-future/ - 0V7xYaT63O2ACftY.99.

200. Wilke, J. *Americans Back Higher Health Insurance Rates for Smokers.* 2013 August 12 [cited 2013 October 10]; Available from: http://www.gallup.com/poll/163925/americans-back-higher-health-insurance-rates-smokers.aspx.

201. Doheny, K. *Smokers and the Affordable Care Act: Q&A.* 2013 August 27 [cited 2013 October 10]; Available from: http://www.webmd.com/health-insurance/20130716/how-affordable-care-act-affects-smokers.

202. Anonymous. *RAND: Workplace Wellness Programs Don't Deliver.* 2013 May 29 [cited 2013 July 20]; Available from: http://www.advisory.com/Daily-Briefing/2013/05/29/RAND-Workplace-wellness-programs-dont-deliver.

203. Anonymous. *From Fitbit to Fitocracy: The Rise of Health Care Gamification.* 2013 January 16 [cited 2013 October 9]; Available from: http://knowledge.wharton.upenn.edu/article/from-fitbit-to-fitocracy-the-rise-of-health-care-gamification/.

204. Comstock, J. *Real Games for Health and the Trouble with Gamification* 2012 December 4 [cited 2013 October 3]; Available from: http://mobihealthnews.com/19323/real-games-for-health-and-the-trouble-with-gamification/.

205. Resnik, D.B. *Charging Smokers Higher Health Insurance Rates: Is it Ethical?* 2013 September 19 [cited 2013 September 23]; Available from: http://www.thehastingscenter.org/Bioethicsforum/Post.aspx?id=6516&blogid=140.

206. Calbucci, M. *Xbox One, Kinect 2.0 and the Future of Health Technology.* 2013 May 26 [cited 2013 June 15]; Available from: http://mobihealthnews.com/22628/.

207. Stone, K. *And So It Begins.* 2004 July 13 [cited 2013 August 27]; Available from: http://www.postpartumprogress.com/author/katherine-stone/page/460.

208. Stone, K. *Postpartum Progress Testimonials.* 2012 [cited 2013 August 27]; Available from: http://www.postpartumprogress.com/testimonials.

209. Anonymous. *Obamacare.* 2013 October 1 [cited 2013 October 15]; Available from: http://www.inspire.com/groups/talk-psoriasis/discussion/obamacare-4/.

210. Anonymous. *Global Rise in Dementia Creates Caregiver Shortage* 2013 September 19 [cited 2013 October 15]; Available from: http://www.voanews.com/content/reu-global-rise-in-dementia-creating-chronic-shortage-of-elderly-caregivers/1753362.html.

211. deBronkart, D. *Gimme My Damn Data: Cancer Patient Xeni Finds a "Ghost Penis" in Her Bone Scan.* 2011 December 20 [cited 2013 September 7]; Available from: http://e-patients.net/archives/2011/12/gimme-my-damn-data-cancer-patient-xeni-finds-a-ghost-penis-in-her-bone-scan.html.

212. Anonymous. *Meaningful Use Definition & Objectives* 2013 [cited 2013 September 3]; Available from: http://www.healthit.gov/providers-

professionals/meaningful-use-definition-objectives.

213. McCartney, Z. *Patient Portal Mandate Triggers Anxiety* Healthcare IT News, August 2, 2013.

214. Pinsker, B. *Electronic Health Records Still Require Manual Labor* Reuters, August 13, 2013.

215. deBronkart, D. *Rookie e-patient @Xeni Helps the Docs View Her Data.* 2011 December 22 [cited 2013 September 6]; Available from: http://e-patients.net/archives/2011/12/rookie-epatient-xeni.html.

216. Anonymous. *Patient Activation Measure.* 2009 [cited 2013 September 29]; Available from: http://www.insigniahealth.com/ha/measure.html.

217. Wilkins, S. *Patient Engagement Is a Physician-Patient Communication Challenge...Not a Health Information Technology Challenge.* 2012 September 12 [cited 2013 September 14]; Available from: http://mindthegap.smarthealthmessaging.com/2012/09/10/patient-engagement-is-a-physician-patient-communication-challenge-not-a-health-information-technology-challenge/.

218. Fox, S., *The Social Life of Health Information, 2011.* 2011, Pew Internet and American Life Project: Washington, DC.

219. Anonymous. *About the Blue Button Movement.* 2013 [cited 2013 October 15]; Available from: http://www.healthit.gov/patients-families/about-blue-button-movement.

220. Hayes, T. *Thoughts on Blue Button: 6 Reasons Why It Lacks Adoption, and Its Troubled Future.* 2013 October 4 [cited 2013 November 7]; Available from: http://electronichealthreporter.com/thoughts-on-blue-button-6-reasons-why-it-lacks-adoption-and-its-troubled-future/.

221. Garrett, P. *Help Us Put Blue Button on the Map.* 2013 September 16 [cited 2013 November 7]; Available from: http://www.healthit.gov/buzz-blog/health-innovation/put-blue-button-map/.

222. Epstein, S., *Impure Science: AIDS, Activism, and the Politics of Knowledge* 1996, Berkeley: University of California Press.

223. Best, R.K., *Disease Politics and Medical Research Funding: Three Ways Advocacy Shapes Policy.* American Sociological Review, 2012. 77(5): p. 780-803.

224. Goldberg, J. *Breakthrough.* 1997 January 12 [cited 2013 September 10]; Available from: http://www.nytimes.com/books/97/01/12/reviews/970112.12goldbet.html.

225. France, D., *How to Survive a Plague.* 2012, Sundance Selects: United States

226. McVicar, N., *AIDS Patients Go Underground for Drug Tests,* in *Florida Sun Sentinel* June 28, 1989.

227. Marcus, A.D., *Frustrated ALS Patients Concoct Their Own Drug* in *Wall*

Street Journal April 15, 2012: New York.

228. Akst, J., *Do-It-Yourself Medicine*, in *The Scientist* March 1, 2013.

229. Anonymous. *Patient Led Funding for Clinical Trials*. 2012 November 15 [cited 2013 September 8]; Available from: http://ecancer.org/conference/159-ncri-2012/video/1724/patient-led-funding-for-clinical-trials.php.

230. Anonymous. *Personal Genome Project: Our Mission*. 2013 [cited 2013 September 8]; Available from: http://www.personalgenomes.org/mission.

231. Gorski, D. *Balancing Scientific Rigor versus Patient Good in Clinical Trials*. 2010 September 20 [cited 2013 September 6]; Available from: http://scienceblogs.com/insolence/2010/09/20/balancing-scientific-rigor-versus-patien/.

232. Swan, M., *Crowdsourced Health Research Studies: An Important Emerging Complement to Clinical Trials in the Public Health Research Ecosystem*. Journal of Medical Internet Research, 2012. **14**(2): p. e46.

233. Skloot, R., *The Immortal Life of Henrietta Lacks* 2010, New York: Crown Publishers.

234. Lewis, D., *Now I Know: The Revealing Stories Behind the World's Most Interesting Facts* 2013, Avon: Adams Media.

235. Anonymous. September 2010 - Health Tracking: Data Set Released by the Pew Research Center 2010 September 1 [cited 2012 March]; Available from: http://pewinternet.org/Shared-Content/Data-Sets/2010/September-2010-Health.aspx.

Acknowledgements

We'd like to take a moment to thank the many people who helped make this book a success.

To those who agreed to participate in interviews for this book—sometimes at the very last minute—Dave deBronkart, Andre Blackman, Bonnie Feldman, Jody Ranck, and Nedra Weinreich.

To Regina Holliday, for giving us permission to use an image from her Walking Gallery in this book.

To Noor Thapa, Enspektos' Chief Technology Officer and certified miracle worker, for his heroic efforts to ensure that digihealth pulse, enmoebius, and other engines of the company's research efforts are operating at peak efficiency.

To the kind people at Health 2.0, Matthew Holt, Kim Krueger, and Prerna Anand, who gave us an opportunity to present *ePatient 2015* to a global audience of health technology enthusiasts and provided a sounding board for some of the ideas in the book.

To Susannah Fox at the Pew Research Center for her nearly 15 years of pioneering research, which laid the groundwork for this book.